AF830893

Demystifying Dit Da

Ancient Wisdom for Modern Healing

Mei Lin Zhang

Xspurts.com

A New Zealand Designed Product

Other Versions Available

Why limit yourself to just one format?

This book is now available in physical, digital, and audiobook options.

Choose the way you love to read and dive into the story today. You won't regret it!

Digital ISBN: 9781776968275
Physical ISBN: 9781776968268
Audio ISBN:

To obtain a different format of this book at a discounted price, please get in touch with us at:

http://isbn.xspurts.com/

Contents

Get Free Stuff

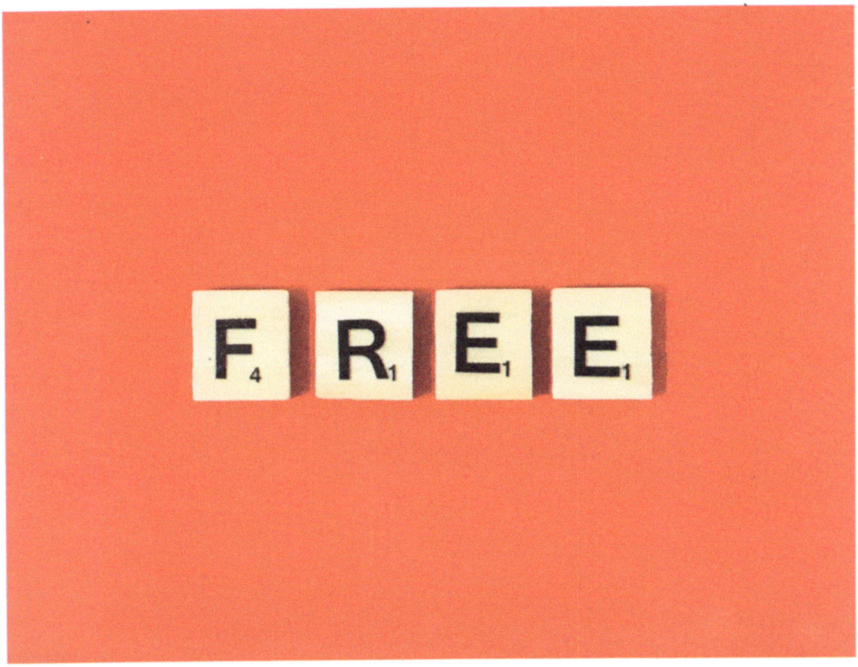

We love writing and have produced a huge number of books.

For being one of our amazing readers, we would love to offer you more books we have created, 100% free.

To claim this limited time special offer, simply go to the site below and enter your name and email address.

You will then receive loads (as we love our readers so much :) of our great books, content and audio direct to your email account, 100% free!

Get Loads of FREE Stuff at:

https://free.xspurts.com

Chapter One

Introduction to Dit Da

Dit Da is a traditional Chinese medicine practice that has been used for centuries to treat injuries and promote healing. The term "Dit Da" literally translates to "hit medicine," reflecting its origins as a method for treating the injuries sustained in martial arts and other physical activities.

Dit Da encompasses a variety of techniques and practices, including herbal medicine, massage, acupuncture, and bone setting. It is based on the principles of Traditional Chinese Medicine (TCM), which views the body as a network of interconnected systems that must be in balance in order to achieve health and well-being.

History of Dit Da

The origins of Dit Da can be traced back to ancient China, where it was practiced by martial artists and warriors as a way to treat injuries sustained in battle. Over time, it became more widely used by the general population as a form of self-care and healing.

One of the earliest written records of Dit Da can be found in the Huangdi Neijing, a classic text on Chinese medicine dating back to the 2nd century BCE. The text describes a variety of techniques for treating injuries, including the use of herbs, massage, and acupuncture.

In the centuries that followed, Dit Da continued to evolve and adapt to new cultural and technological changes. During the Ming Dynasty

(1368-1644), for example, Dit Da practitioners began using bone-setting techniques to realign broken or dislocated bones.

By the Qing Dynasty (1644-1912), Dit Da had become an established branch of Chinese medicine, with its own specialized practitioners and techniques.

Principles of Dit Da

At the heart of Dit Da is the principle of qi, the vital energy that flows through the body and animates all life. According to TCM, injuries and illnesses are caused by imbalances or blockages in the flow of qi, which can be corrected through various techniques and practices.

In Dit Da, the goal is to restore the flow of qi and promote the body's natural healing processes. This is done through a combination of herbal medicine, massage, acupuncture, and other techniques, all tailored to the individual needs of the patient.

Herbal Medicine

Herbal medicine is a central component of Dit Da, and a wide variety of herbs are used to treat injuries and promote healing. These herbs are often combined into formulas that are tailored to the specific needs of the patient.

Some of the most commonly used herbs in Dit Da include:

1. Dang Gui: a root that is used to promote blood circulation and relieve pain

2. Huang Qin: a root that has anti-inflammatory and antibacterial properties

3. Fang Feng: a root that is used to relieve pain and promote healing

4. Gan Cao: a root that is used to calm the mind and relieve pain

5. Hong Hua: a flower that is used to promote blood circulation and relieve pain

Massage

Massage is another important component of Dit Da, and is used to promote the flow of qi and relieve pain and tension in the muscles and other soft tissues. There are many different massage techniques used in Dit Da, each with its own specific benefits and applications.

Some of the most common massage techniques used in Dit Da include:

6. Tui Na: a form of Chinese therapeutic massage that uses a variety of techniques to stimulate the flow of qi and relieve pain and tension

7. Gua Sha: a scraping technique that is used to promote blood circulation and relieve pain

8. Cupping: a technique that uses suction to stimulate the flow of qi and relieve pain and tension

Acupuncture

Acupuncture is a key component of TCM, and is used in Dit Da to promote the flow of qi and relieve pain and tension in the body. Acupuncture involves the insertion of thin needles into specific points on the body, known as acupoints.

The history and origins of

Dit

Da

Dit Da is a traditional Chinese medicine practice that has been used for centuries to treat injuries and promote healing. The term "Dit Da" literally translates to "hit medicine," reflecting its origins as a method for treating the injuries sustained in martial arts and other physical activities.

The history of Dit Da can be traced back to ancient China, where it was practiced by martial artists and warriors as a way to treat injuries sustained in battle. Over time, it became more widely used by the general population as a form of self-care and healing.

One of the earliest written records of Dit Da can be found in the Huangdi Neijing, a classic text on Chinese medicine dating back to the 2nd century BCE. The text describes a variety of techniques for treating injuries, including the use of herbs, massage, and acupuncture.

During the Han Dynasty (206 BCE - 220 CE), Dit Da began to emerge as a distinct branch of Chinese medicine, with its own specialized practitioners and techniques. This was due in part to the popularity of martial arts during this time period, which led to an increased need for effective methods of treating injuries.

One of the most famous early practitioners of Dit Da was Hua Tuo, a legendary physician who lived during the late Han Dynasty. Hua Tuo is credited with developing a number of innovative techniques for treating injuries, including the use of anesthetic herbal preparations and surgical procedures.

During the Tang Dynasty (618-907 CE), Dit Da continued to evolve and develop, with many new techniques and practices being introduced. It was during this time that bone-setting techniques began to be used to realign broken or dislocated bones.

By the Song Dynasty (960-1279 CE), Dit Da had become an established branch of Chinese medicine, with its own specialized practitioners and techniques. During this time, the focus of Dit Da shifted from treating injuries sustained in battle to treating injuries sustained in everyday life.

One of the most famous practitioners of Dit Da during the Song Dynasty was Sun Simiao, a physician and scholar who is often referred to as the "King of Medicine." Sun Simiao was known for his expertise in herbal medicine and his commitment to treating all patients, regardless of their social status or ability to pay.

During the Ming Dynasty (1368-1644), Dit Da continued to evolve and adapt to new cultural and technological changes. This was a time of great social and cultural change in China, and Dit Da practitioners were at the forefront of many of these changes.

One of the most significant developments in Dit Da during the Ming Dynasty was the use of bone-setting techniques to realign broken or dislocated bones. This technique was known as "Zheng Gu," and was developed by the famous physician and martial artist Wong Fei Hung.

During the Qing Dynasty (1644-1912), Dit Da had become an established branch of Chinese medicine, with its own specialized practitioners and techniques. It was during this time that Dit Da began to spread to other parts of the world, as Chinese immigrants brought their knowledge and practices with them.

Today, Dit Da continues to be an important part of Chinese medicine, and is widely used to treat injuries and promote healing. While many of the techniques and practices used in Dit Da have evolved over time, the underlying principles of Traditional Chinese Medicine remain the same, emphasizing the importance of balance and harmony in the body.

The principles of

Dit

Da

At the heart of Dit Da is the principle of qi, the vital energy that flows through the body and animates all life. According to Traditional Chinese Medicine (TCM), injuries and illnesses are caused by imbalances or blockages in the flow of qi, which can be corrected through various techniques and practices.

In Dit Da, the goal is to restore the flow of qi and promote the body's natural healing processes. This is done through a combination of herbal medicine, massage, acupuncture, and other techniques, all tailored to the individual needs of the patient.

Herbal Medicine

Herbal medicine is a central component of Dit Da, and a wide variety of herbs are used to treat injuries and promote healing. These herbs are often combined into formulas that are tailored to the specific needs of the patient.

Some of the most commonly used herbs in Dit Da include:

1. Dang Gui: a root that is used to promote blood circulation and relieve pain

2. Huang Qin: a root that has anti-inflammatory and antibacterial properties

3. Fang Feng: a root that is used to relieve pain and promote healing

4. Gan Cao: a root that is used to calm the mind and relieve pain

5. Hong Hua: a flower that is used to promote blood circulation and relieve pain

Massage

Massage is another important component of Dit Da, and is used to promote the flow of qi and relieve pain and tension in the muscles and other soft tissues. There are many different massage techniques used in Dit Da, each with its own specific benefits and applications.

Some of the most common massage techniques used in Dit Da include:

6. Tui Na: a form of Chinese therapeutic massage that uses a variety of techniques to stimulate the flow of qi and relieve pain and tension

7. Gua Sha: a scraping technique that is used to promote blood circulation and relieve pain

8. Cupping: a technique that uses suction to stimulate the flow of qi and relieve pain and tension

Acupuncture

Acupuncture is a key component of TCM, and is used in Dit Da to promote the flow of qi and relieve pain and tension in the body. Acupuncture involves the insertion of thin needles into specific points on the body, known as acupoints.

These acupoints are believed to correspond to different organs and systems in the body, and by stimulating them, the flow of qi can be restored and imbalances corrected. Acupuncture is often used in conjunction with other techniques, such as herbal medicine and massage, to provide a comprehensive approach to healing.

Diet and Lifestyle

In addition to herbal medicine, massage, and acupuncture, diet and lifestyle also play an important role in Dit Da. According to TCM, what we eat and how we live can have a profound impact on our health and well-being.

In Dit Da, patients are often advised to eat a healthy, balanced diet that includes a variety of fresh fruits and vegetables, whole grains, and lean proteins. They may also be advised to avoid certain foods that can exacerbate their condition, such as spicy or greasy foods.

In addition to dietary changes, lifestyle modifications may also be recommended. This may include getting more exercise, practicing stress-reduction techniques such as meditation or tai chi, and getting adequate rest and sleep.

Chapter Two

Understanding Dit Da Medicine

Dit Da is a traditional Chinese medicine practice that has been used for centuries to treat injuries and promote healing. The term "Dit Da" literally translates to "hit medicine," reflecting its origins as a method for treating the injuries sustained in martial arts and other physical activities. Today, Dit Da is widely used to treat a variety of injuries and ailments, and is an important part of Traditional Chinese Medicine (TCM).

The Principles of Dit Da

At the heart of Dit Da is the principle of qi, the vital energy that flows through the body and animates all life. According to TCM, injuries and illnesses are caused by imbalances or blockages in the flow of qi, which can be corrected through various techniques and practices.

In Dit Da, the goal is to restore the flow of qi and promote the body's natural healing processes. This is done through a combination of herbal medicine, massage, acupuncture, and other techniques, all tailored to the individual needs of the patient.

Herbal Medicine in Dit Da

Herbal medicine is a central component of Dit Da, and a wide variety of herbs are used to treat injuries and promote healing. These herbs are often combined into formulas that are tailored to the specific needs of the patient.

Some of the most commonly used herbs in Dit Da include:

1. Dang Gui: a root that is used to promote blood circulation and relieve pain

2. Huang Qin: a root that has anti-inflammatory and antibacterial properties

3. Fang Feng: a root that is used to relieve pain and promote healing

4. Gan Cao: a root that is used to calm the mind and relieve pain

5. Hong Hua: a flower that is used to promote blood circulation and relieve pain

Massage Techniques in Dit Da

Massage is another important component of Dit Da, and is used to promote the flow of qi and relieve pain and tension in the muscles and other soft tissues. There are many different massage techniques used in Dit Da, each with its own specific benefits and applications.

Some of the most common massage techniques used in Dit Da include:

6. Tui Na: a form of Chinese therapeutic massage that uses a variety of techniques to stimulate the flow of qi and relieve pain and tension

7. Gua Sha: a scraping technique that is used to promote blood circulation and relieve pain

8. Cupping: a technique that uses suction to stimulate the flow of qi and relieve pain and tension

Acupuncture in Dit Da

Acupuncture is a key component of TCM, and is used in Dit Da to promote the flow of qi and relieve pain and tension in the body. Acupuncture involves the insertion of thin needles into specific points on the body, known as acupoints.

These acupoints are believed to correspond to different organs and systems in the body, and by stimulating them, the flow of qi can be restored and imbalances corrected. Acupuncture is often used in conjunction with other techniques, such as herbal medicine and massage, to provide a comprehensive approach to healing.

Diet and Lifestyle in Dit Da

In addition to herbal medicine, massage, and acupuncture, diet and lifestyle also play an important role in Dit Da. According to TCM, what we eat and how we live can have a profound impact on our health and well-being.

In Dit Da, patients are often advised to eat a healthy, balanced diet that includes a variety of fresh fruits and vegetables, whole grains, and lean proteins. They may also be advised to avoid certain foods that can exacerbate their condition, such as spicy or greasy foods.

In addition to dietary changes, lifestyle modifications may also be recommended. This may include getting more exercise, practicing stress-reduction techniques such as meditation or tai chi, and getting adequate rest and sleep.

The role of Chinese herbs in

Dit

Da

Chinese herbs have been used for centuries in traditional Chinese medicine practices such as Dit Da. These herbs are believed to have therapeutic properties that can help to promote healing and restore balance in the body. In Dit Da, Chinese herbs are often used in combination with other techniques such as massage and acupuncture to treat injuries and promote overall health and well-being.

Types of Chinese Herbs Used in Dit Da

There are many different types of Chinese herbs that are used in Dit Da. Some of the most commonly used herbs include:

1. Dang Gui: This herb is commonly used to promote blood circulation and relieve pain. It is often used to treat injuries such as bruises and sprains.

2. Huang Qin: This herb has anti-inflammatory and antibacterial properties, making it useful for treating infections and inflammation.

3. Fang Feng: This herb is known for its ability to relieve pain and promote healing. It is often used to treat injuries such as fractures and dislocations.

4. Gan Cao: This herb is used to calm the mind and relieve pain. It is often used to treat injuries such as strains and sprains.

5. Hong Hua: This herb is used to promote blood circulation and relieve pain. It is often used to treat injuries such as bruises and contusions.

Other herbs that may be used in Dit Da include Dang Shen, Bai Zhi, Gui Zhi, and Chuan Xiong.

Preparation and Administration of Chinese Herbs in Dit Da

Chinese herbs used in Dit Da are often prepared in the form of herbal formulas. These formulas may be prepared as a tea or decoction, or in the form of pills or powders. The specific formula used will depend on the individual needs of the patient and the nature of their injury or condition.

In some cases, Chinese herbs may also be applied topically in the form of a liniment or ointment. These preparations may be made by steeping the herbs in a carrier oil, such as sesame oil or alcohol, and then applying the resulting mixture to the affected area.

Safety Considerations

While Chinese herbs used in Dit Da are generally considered safe when used appropriately, it is important to exercise caution when using these remedies. Some herbs may interact with medications or have potential side effects, particularly if used in large doses or for prolonged periods of time.

For this reason, it is important to consult with a qualified practitioner of traditional Chinese medicine before using any herbal remedies. They can help to assess your individual needs and develop a treatment plan that is safe and effective.

Balancing yin and yang in

Dit

Da medicine

Dit Da is a traditional Chinese medicine practice that has been used for centuries to treat injuries and promote healing. At the heart of Dit Da is the principle of balance, and the importance of balancing the opposing forces of yin and yang in the body.

Understanding Yin and Yang in TCM

In Traditional Chinese Medicine (TCM), the concept of yin and yang is central to understanding health and disease. Yin and yang are opposing forces that are present in all things, including the human body. Yin represents the more passive, receptive, and cooling aspects of nature, while yang represents the more active, dynamic, and warming aspects of nature.

According to TCM, health and well-being depend on a delicate balance between these opposing forces. When yin and yang are in balance, the body is able to function optimally and resist disease. However, when yin and yang are imbalanced, this can lead to illness and a range of health problems.

Balancing Yin and Yang in Dit Da

In Dit Da, the goal is to restore balance to the body by balancing the opposing forces of yin and yang. This is done through a combination of techniques and practices, including herbal medicine, massage, acupuncture, and lifestyle modifications.

Herbal Medicine

Herbal medicine is a key component of Dit Da, and is often used to restore balance to the body by addressing imbalances in yin and yang. For example, if a patient has a condition that is characterized by excess heat and inflammation, cooling herbs may be prescribed to restore balance and bring yin and yang into harmony.

Some of the most commonly used herbs in Dit Da for balancing yin and yang include:

1. Huang Qin: This herb has a cooling and drying effect and is often used to clear excess heat and inflammation from the body.

2. Dang Gui: This herb has a nourishing and warming effect and is often used to promote blood circulation and strengthen the body's qi.

3. Gan Cao: This herb has a harmonizing effect and is often used to balance the actions of other herbs in an herbal formula.

Massage Techniques

Massage is another important component of Dit Da and is used to balance yin and yang by promoting the flow of qi and blood. Different massage techniques may be used depending on the individual needs of the patient.

For example, Tui Na massage is often used to stimulate the flow of qi and blood in areas of stagnation or blockage, while Gua Sha is often used to promote blood circulation and relieve pain.

Acupuncture

Acupuncture is also used in Dit Da to balance yin and yang by stimulating the flow of qi and blood. Specific acupuncture points may be used depending on the individual needs of the patient and the nature of their injury or condition.

For example, if a patient has a condition that is characterized by excess heat and inflammation, acupuncture points that have a cooling and calming effect may be used to restore balance.

Diet and Lifestyle Modifications

In addition to herbal medicine, massage, and acupuncture, diet and lifestyle modifications may also be recommended in Dit Da to balance yin and yang. This may include recommendations for dietary changes, exercise, and stress-reduction techniques such as meditation or tai chi.

For example, if a patient has a condition that is characterized by excess heat and inflammation, they may be advised to avoid spicy or greasy foods and to incorporate more cooling and hydrating foods into their diet.

Chapter Three

The Art of Bone Setting

Bone setting is a traditional medical practice that has been used for centuries to treat musculoskeletal injuries and conditions. Also known as orthopedic manual therapy, bone setting is a manual technique that involves manipulating the bones, joints, and soft tissues to promote healing and restore proper function.

In traditional Chinese medicine practices such as Dit Da, bone setting is often used in conjunction with other techniques such as herbal medicine, acupuncture, and massage to provide a comprehensive approach to healing.

History of Bone Setting

The history of bone setting can be traced back to ancient civilizations such as Egypt and Greece, where it was used to treat musculoskeletal injuries and conditions. In China, bone setting has been practiced for thousands of years and is a key component of traditional Chinese medicine.

Bone setting was traditionally practiced by specialized practitioners known as bone setters, who were skilled in manipulating the bones, joints, and soft tissues to promote healing. Over time, bone setting has become more standardized and is now often performed by licensed medical practitioners such as osteopaths and chiropractors.

Techniques of Bone Setting

Bone setting involves a range of techniques and approaches, depending on the nature and severity of the injury or condition. Some of the most common techniques used in bone setting include:

1. Joint manipulation: This involves the gentle manipulation of a joint to restore proper alignment and range of motion.

2. Soft tissue mobilization: This involves the manipulation of the soft tissues, such as muscles, tendons, and ligaments, to promote healing and restore proper function.

3. Traction: This involves the application of gentle pulling forces to the bones and joints to relieve pressure and promote healing.

4. Massage: This involves the application of pressure and friction to the soft tissues to promote blood flow and reduce pain and stiffness.

Bone setting may also involve the use of specialized tools such as traction devices, braces, and splints to support the injured area and promote healing.

Benefits of Bone Setting

Bone setting can provide a range of benefits for individuals with musculoskeletal injuries and conditions. Some of the most common benefits of bone setting include:

5. Pain relief: By manipulating the bones and soft tissues, bone setting can help to relieve pain and discomfort associated with musculoskeletal injuries and conditions.

6. Improved range of motion: By restoring proper alignment and function to the bones and joints, bone setting can help to improve range of motion and mobility.

7. Faster healing: By promoting blood flow and reducing pressure on the injured area, bone setting can help to promote faster healing and recovery.

8. Non-invasive: Bone setting is a non-invasive approach to treating musculoskeletal injuries and conditions, and does not involve the use of drugs or surgery.

Precautions and Considerations

While bone setting is generally considered safe when performed by a qualified practitioner, there are some precautions and considerations that should be taken into account. In some cases, bone setting may not be appropriate or may need to be modified depending on the individual needs of the patient.

For example, individuals with certain medical conditions such as osteoporosis or arthritis may need to avoid certain techniques or modifications may need to be made to accommodate their condition. It is important to consult with a qualified practitioner of bone setting to determine the most appropriate approach for your individual needs.

The importance of bone alignment

Proper bone alignment is essential for maintaining optimal health and function in the body. When bones are misaligned, it can cause a range of problems such as pain, stiffness, and limited mobility. In traditional Chinese medicine practices such as Dit Da, the importance of bone alignment is emphasized, and techniques such as bone setting are used to promote proper alignment and restore function.

What is Bone Alignment?

Bone alignment refers to the proper positioning of the bones in the body. This is essential for maintaining proper function and mobility, as well as preventing injuries and conditions such as arthritis and osteoporosis.

When bones are misaligned, it can cause pressure on surrounding tissues and joints, leading to pain, inflammation, and reduced mobility. Misalignments can occur as a result of injuries, poor posture, or underlying medical conditions.

The Importance of Bone Alignment in Dit Da

In Dit Da, the importance of bone alignment is emphasized, and techniques such as bone setting are used to promote proper alignment and restore function. Bone setting is a manual technique that involves manipulating the bones and soft tissues to promote healing and restore proper alignment.

By restoring proper alignment, bone setting can help to relieve pain and stiffness, improve range of motion and mobility, and promote overall health and well-being. This is achieved by realigning the bones and joints to their proper position, relieving pressure on surrounding tissues, and promoting proper function and movement.

Techniques Used in Bone Setting

Bone setting involves a range of techniques and approaches, depending on the nature and severity of the injury or condition. Some of the most common techniques used in bone setting include:

1. Joint manipulation: This involves the gentle manipulation of a joint to restore proper alignment and range of motion.

2. Soft tissue mobilization: This involves the manipulation of the soft tissues, such as muscles, tendons, and ligaments, to promote healing and restore proper function.

3. Traction: This involves the application of gentle pulling forces to the bones and joints to relieve pressure and promote healing.

4. Massage: This involves the application of pressure and friction to the soft tissues to promote blood flow and reduce pain and stiffness.

Bone setting may also involve the use of specialized tools such as traction devices, braces, and splints to support the injured area and promote healing.

Benefits of Proper Bone Alignment

Proper bone alignment can provide a range of benefits for individuals, including:

5. Reduced pain and stiffness: By relieving pressure on surrounding tissues and joints, proper bone alignment can help to reduce pain and stiffness associated with musculoskeletal injuries and conditions.

6. Improved range of motion: By restoring proper alignment and function to the bones and joints, proper bone alignment can help to improve range of motion and mobility.

7. Enhanced athletic performance: Proper bone alignment can help to improve athletic performance by reducing the risk of injury and improving overall function and mobility.

8. Improved overall health and well-being: Proper bone alignment is essential for maintaining overall health and well-being, as misalignments can lead to a range of problems and conditions.

Common techniques for bone setting

Bone setting is a traditional medical practice that has been used for centuries to treat musculoskeletal injuries and conditions. Also known as orthopedic manual therapy, bone setting involves manipulating the bones, joints, and soft tissues to promote healing and restore proper function. In traditional Chinese medicine practices such as Dit Da, bone setting is often used in conjunction with other techniques such as herbal medicine, acupuncture, and massage to provide a comprehensive approach to healing.

There are several common techniques used in bone setting, each with its own unique benefits and applications. Here are some of the most commonly used techniques:

Joint Manipulation

Joint manipulation is a technique that involves the gentle manipulation of a joint to restore proper alignment and range of motion. This technique is often used to treat conditions such as joint stiffness, restricted mobility, and musculoskeletal pain.

Joint manipulation works by applying a controlled force to the joint, which causes it to move beyond its normal range of motion. This movement can help to loosen tight muscles and tissues surrounding the joint, and can also stimulate the production of synovial fluid, which helps to lubricate the joint and improve its function.

Soft Tissue Mobilization

Soft tissue mobilization is a technique that involves the manipulation of the soft tissues, such as muscles, tendons, and ligaments, to promote healing and restore proper function. This technique is often used to treat conditions such as sprains, strains, and musculoskeletal pain.

Soft tissue mobilization works by applying pressure to the soft tissues using various techniques such as kneading, squeezing, and stretching. This pressure can help to increase blood flow to the affected area, which can promote healing and reduce pain and stiffness.

Traction

Traction is a technique that involves the application of gentle pulling forces to the bones and joints to relieve pressure and promote healing. This technique is often used to treat conditions such as herniated discs, sciatica, and spinal stenosis.

Traction works by decompressing the affected area, which can help to relieve pressure on the nerves and tissues surrounding the affected area. This can reduce pain and improve overall function and mobility.

Massage

Massage is a technique that involves the application of pressure and friction to the soft tissues to promote blood flow and reduce pain and stiffness. This technique is often used to treat conditions such as muscle spasms, tension headaches, and musculoskeletal pain.

Massage works by stimulating the production of endorphins, which are natural painkillers produced by the body. Massage can also help to reduce muscle tension and improve blood flow, which can promote healing and reduce pain and stiffness.

Acupuncture

Acupuncture is a technique that involves the insertion of thin needles into specific points on the body to stimulate healing and restore proper function. This technique is often used to treat conditions such as chronic pain, arthritis, and musculoskeletal injuries.

Acupuncture works by stimulating the flow of energy, or qi, in the body. By inserting needles into specific points, acupuncturists can help to balance the flow of qi and promote healing and restoration of proper function.

Chapter Four

Dit Da and Martial Arts

Dit Da is a traditional Chinese medicine practice that has been used for centuries to treat musculoskeletal injuries and conditions. Also known as "hit medicine," Dit Da is often used in conjunction with martial arts practices to help athletes recover from injuries and improve their performance.

History of Dit Da in Martial Arts

The use of Dit Da in martial arts can be traced back to ancient China, where martial artists often suffered from injuries such as bruises, sprains, and fractures as a result of their training. To aid in their recovery, these martial artists turned to Dit Da, which proved to be an effective treatment for their injuries.

Over time, Dit Da became a central part of martial arts practices, and many martial arts schools began to develop their own unique formulas and techniques for using Dit Da to improve performance and prevent injuries.

How Dit Da is Used in Martial Arts

Dit Da is often used in martial arts practices to help athletes recover from injuries and improve their performance. Some of the ways that Dit Da is used in martial arts include:

1. Treating injuries: Dit Da is often used to treat injuries such as bruises, sprains, and fractures that can occur during martial arts training.

2. Preventing injuries: By improving circulation and promoting healing, Dit Da can help to prevent injuries from occurring in the first place.

3. Improving performance: By promoting healing and reducing pain and stiffness, Dit Da can help athletes to improve their performance and mobility.

4. Supporting overall health: Dit Da is also used to support overall health and well-being, helping athletes to recover from injuries and maintain optimal health and function.

Techniques Used in Dit Da for Martial Arts

There are several common techniques used in Dit Da for martial arts, each with its own unique benefits and applications. These techniques include:

5. Bone setting: Bone setting is a manual technique that involves manipulating the bones and soft tissues to promote healing and restore proper function. This technique is often used to treat injuries such as fractures and dislocations.

6. Cupping: Cupping is a technique that involves the use of suction cups to promote blood flow and reduce pain and stiffness. This technique is often used to treat injuries such as sprains and strains.

7. Herbal medicine: Herbal medicine is often used in conjunction with other techniques to promote healing and improve overall health and well-being.

8. Acupuncture: Acupuncture is a technique that involves the insertion of thin needles into specific points on the body to stimulate healing and restore proper function. This technique is often used to treat conditions such as chronic pain and musculoskeletal injuries.

Benefits of Dit Da in Martial Arts

Dit Da can provide a range of benefits for athletes practicing martial arts, including:

9. Reduced pain and stiffness: By promoting healing and reducing inflammation, Dit Da can help to reduce pain and stiffness associated with musculoskeletal injuries and conditions.

10. Improved range of motion: By restoring proper alignment and function to the bones and joints, Dit Da can help to improve range of motion and mobility.

11. Faster healing: By promoting blood flow and reducing pressure on the injured area, Dit Da can help to promote faster healing and recovery.

12. Improved overall health and well-being: By supporting overall health and well-being, Dit Da can help athletes to recover from injuries and maintain optimal health and function.

The relationship between

Dit

Da and Kung Fu

Dit Da, a traditional Chinese medicine practice, has been used for centuries to treat musculoskeletal injuries and conditions. One of the primary practices that have used Dit Da is Kung Fu, a Chinese martial art that has been practiced for thousands of years. The relationship between Dit Da and Kung Fu is a strong one, as Kung Fu practitioners often turn to Dit Da to help them recover from injuries and improve their performance.

History of Dit Da and Kung Fu

The use of Dit Da in Kung Fu can be traced back to ancient China, where martial artists often suffered from injuries such as bruises, sprains, and fractures as a result of their training. To aid in their recovery, these martial artists turned to Dit Da, which proved to be an effective treatment for their injuries.

Over time, the use of Dit Da became an integral part of Kung Fu practices, with many Kung Fu schools developing their own unique formulas and techniques for using Dit Da to improve performance and prevent injuries.

How Dit Da is Used in Kung Fu

Dit Da is often used in Kung Fu practices to help athletes recover from injuries and improve their performance. Some of the ways that Dit Da is used in Kung Fu include:

1. Treating injuries: Dit Da is often used to treat injuries such as bruises, sprains, and fractures that can occur during Kung Fu training.

2. Preventing injuries: By improving circulation and promoting healing, Dit Da can help to prevent injuries from occurring in the first place.

3. Improving performance: By promoting healing and reducing pain and stiffness, Dit Da can help athletes to improve their performance and mobility.

4. Supporting overall health: Dit Da is also used to support overall health and well-being, helping athletes to recover from injuries and maintain optimal health and function.

Techniques Used in Dit Da for Kung Fu

There are several common techniques used in Dit Da for Kung Fu, each with its own unique benefits and applications. These techniques include:

5. Bone setting: Bone setting is a manual technique that involves manipulating the bones and soft tissues to promote healing and restore proper function. This technique is often used to treat injuries such as fractures and dislocations.

6. Cupping: Cupping is a technique that involves the use of suction cups to promote blood flow and reduce pain and stiffness. This technique is often used to treat injuries such as sprains and strains.

7. Herbal medicine: Herbal medicine is often used in conjunction with other techniques to promote healing and improve overall health and well-being.

8. Acupuncture: Acupuncture is a technique that involves the insertion of thin needles into specific points on the body to stimulate healing and restore proper function. This technique is often used to treat conditions such as chronic pain and musculoskeletal injuries.

Benefits of Dit Da in Kung Fu

Dit Da can provide a range of benefits for athletes practicing Kung Fu, including:

9. Reduced pain and stiffness: By promoting healing and reducing inflammation, Dit Da can help to reduce pain and stiffness associated with musculoskeletal injuries and conditions.

10. Improved range of motion: By restoring proper alignment and function to the bones and joints, Dit Da can help to improve range of motion and mobility.

11. Faster healing: By promoting blood flow and reducing pressure on the injured area, Dit Da can help to promote faster healing and recovery.

12. Improved overall health and well-being: By supporting overall health and well-being, Dit Da can help athletes to recover from injuries and maintain optimal health and function.

Injury prevention and recovery in martial arts

Martial arts is a physically demanding sport that requires athletes to push their bodies to the limit. As a result, injuries are a common occurrence in martial arts, and athletes need to take steps to prevent injuries and promote recovery. One traditional Chinese medicine practice that can aid in this process is Dit Da.

Dit Da is a practice that has been used for centuries to treat musculoskeletal injuries and conditions. In martial arts practices, Dit Da is often used to help athletes recover from injuries and improve their performance. Here are some ways that Dit Da can help with injury prevention and recovery in martial arts.

Preventing Injuries

One of the primary ways that Dit Da can help with injury prevention is by promoting proper alignment and function of the bones and joints. By using techniques such as bone setting and cupping, Dit Da can help to reduce the risk of injuries such as sprains, strains, and fractures.

Bone setting involves manipulating the bones and soft tissues to promote healing and restore proper function. This technique can help to prevent injuries by ensuring that the bones and joints are properly aligned and functioning as they should.

Cupping is a technique that involves the use of suction cups to promote blood flow and reduce pain and stiffness. This technique can help to prevent injuries by improving circulation and reducing tension in the muscles and soft tissues.

Improving Recovery

When injuries do occur, Dit Da can also help athletes to recover more quickly and effectively. By promoting blood flow and reducing inflammation, Dit Da can help to speed up the healing process and reduce pain and stiffness associated with injuries.

Acupuncture is one technique used in Dit Da that can be particularly effective for injury recovery. By stimulating the flow of energy, or qi, in the body, acupuncture can help to promote healing and reduce pain and inflammation associated with injuries.

Herbal medicine is another aspect of Dit Da that can be helpful for injury recovery. Many traditional Chinese herbs have anti-inflammatory and pain-relieving properties that can aid in the healing process and reduce discomfort associated with injuries.

Supporting Overall Health and Well-Being

In addition to preventing injuries and aiding in recovery, Dit Da can also support overall health and well-being. By promoting proper alignment and function of the bones and joints, Dit Da can help to improve overall mobility and reduce the risk of injuries.

Herbal medicine used in Dit Da can also support overall health by improving digestion, boosting the immune system, and reducing stress and anxiety. These benefits can help athletes to maintain optimal health and function, reducing the risk of injuries and aiding in recovery from injuries when they do occur.

Chapter Five

The Practice of Tui Na

Tui Na is a form of Chinese therapeutic massage that has been used for thousands of years to treat a wide range of musculoskeletal and internal conditions. The practice involves the use of various massage techniques, including kneading, pressing, and tapping, to promote healing and improve overall health and well-being.

Tui Na is closely related to Dit Da, a traditional Chinese medicine practice that is often used in conjunction with martial arts training. In fact, Tui Na is often used as a complement to Dit Da to aid in the treatment of musculoskeletal injuries and conditions.

History of Tui Na

Tui Na can be traced back to ancient China, where it was first developed as a form of manual therapy to treat musculoskeletal and internal conditions. Over time, the practice evolved to include various massage techniques, including kneading, pressing, and tapping.

Today, Tui Na is practiced all over the world, with many practitioners using the techniques to promote healing and improve overall health and well-being.

How Tui Na is Used

Tui Na is used to treat a wide range of musculoskeletal and internal conditions, including:

Back pain

Neck pain

Headaches

Digestive disorders

Respiratory conditions

Sports injuries

The practice is often used in conjunction with other traditional Chinese medicine practices, such as acupuncture and herbal medicine, to provide a comprehensive approach to healing and wellness.

Techniques Used in Tui Na

Tui Na involves the use of various massage techniques to promote healing and improve overall health and well-being. Some of the techniques used in Tui Na include:

1. Kneading: Kneading involves using the fingers and palms to apply pressure to the muscles and soft tissues, promoting relaxation and improving circulation.

2. Pressing: Pressing involves applying pressure to specific points on the body to stimulate the flow of energy, or qi, and promote healing.

3. Tapping: Tapping involves using the fingertips to tap lightly on the muscles and soft tissues, promoting relaxation and improving circulation.

Benefits of Tui Na

Tui Na can provide a range of benefits for individuals seeking to improve their overall health and well-being, including:

4. Reduced pain and stiffness: By promoting healing and reducing inflammation, Tui Na can help to reduce pain and stiffness associated with musculoskeletal conditions.

5. Improved range of motion: By promoting proper alignment and function of the bones and joints, Tui Na can help to improve range of motion and mobility.

6. Improved digestion: By stimulating the flow of energy in the body, Tui Na can help to improve digestion and reduce symptoms of digestive disorders.

7. Reduced stress and anxiety: By promoting relaxation and reducing tension in the muscles and soft tissues, Tui Na can help to reduce stress and anxiety.

Principles of Tui Na massage

Tui Na massage is a form of traditional Chinese medicine that has been used for thousands of years to promote healing and improve overall health and well-being. The practice involves the use of various massage techniques, including kneading, pressing, and tapping, to stimulate the flow of energy, or qi, in the body and promote healing.

Tui Na massage is closely related to Dit Da, a traditional Chinese medicine practice that is often used in conjunction with martial arts training. In fact, Tui Na massage is often used as a complement to Dit Da to aid in the treatment of musculoskeletal injuries and conditions.

Here are some principles of Tui Na massage and how they relate to the practice of Dit Da.

Qi and the Meridian System

One of the primary principles of Tui Na massage is the concept of qi, or energy, and the meridian system through which it flows. In traditional Chinese medicine, it is believed that the body is composed of various channels, or meridians, through which qi flows.

Tui Na massage is based on the principle that stimulating the flow of qi through the meridian system can promote healing and improve overall health and well-being. This principle is closely related to the practice of Dit Da, which also seeks to stimulate the flow of energy in the body to aid in the healing process.

Manipulating Soft Tissues

Another principle of Tui Na massage is the manipulation of soft tissues, including muscles, tendons, and ligaments. The practice involves using various massage techniques to manipulate these soft tissues and promote healing.

Tui Na massage can be particularly effective for treating musculoskeletal conditions, such as sprains, strains, and other injuries. This principle is closely related to the practice of Dit Da, which also involves manipulating soft tissues to aid in the healing process.

The Use of Acupoints

Tui Na massage also involves the use of acupoints, or specific points on the body that are believed to correspond to various organs and systems in the body. By stimulating these acupoints, Tui Na massage can help to promote healing and improve overall health and well-being.

This principle is closely related to the practice of acupuncture, which also involves the use of acupoints to stimulate the flow of qi in the body. Acupuncture is often used in conjunction with Tui Na massage to provide a comprehensive approach to healing and wellness.

Stimulating Blood Flow

Finally, Tui Na massage seeks to stimulate blood flow in the body to promote healing and reduce pain and stiffness. By improving circulation, Tui Na massage can help to reduce inflammation and promote healing in the affected area.

This principle is closely related to the practice of Dit Da, which also seeks to promote blood flow in the body to aid in the healing process.

Techniques for Tui Na application in

Dit

Da

Tui Na is a traditional Chinese medicine practice that involves the use of various massage techniques to promote healing and improve overall health and well-being. In martial arts training, Tui Na is often used in conjunction with Dit Da to aid in the treatment of musculoskeletal injuries and conditions. Here are some techniques for Tui Na application in Dit Da.

Soft Tissue Manipulation

One of the primary techniques used in Tui Na application in Dit Da is soft tissue manipulation. This involves using various massage techniques, including kneading, pressing, and tapping, to manipulate the soft tissues, including muscles, tendons, and ligaments, to promote healing and reduce pain and stiffness.

Soft tissue manipulation can be particularly effective for treating musculoskeletal injuries and conditions, such as sprains, strains, and other soft tissue injuries. By manipulating the soft tissues, Tui Na can help to reduce inflammation, improve circulation, and promote healing in the affected area.

Acupressure

Another technique used in Tui Na application in Dit Da is acupressure, which involves the use of pressure on specific points on the body to stimulate the flow of energy, or qi, and promote healing. Acupressure is similar to acupuncture, but instead of using needles, pressure is applied to the acupoints using the fingers or other tools.

Acupressure can be particularly effective for treating musculoskeletal injuries and conditions, as well as internal conditions such as digestive disorders and respiratory conditions. By stimulating the flow of qi, acupressure can help to reduce pain and inflammation, improve circulation, and promote healing.

Cupping

Cupping is another technique used in Tui Na application in Dit Da. This technique involves the use of suction cups to promote blood flow and reduce pain and stiffness. The cups are placed on the skin and then suctioned to create a vacuum. This technique can be particularly effective for treating musculoskeletal injuries and conditions, as well as respiratory conditions and digestive disorders.

Cupping can help to reduce pain and inflammation, improve circulation, and promote healing in the affected area. It can also help to reduce tension in the muscles and soft tissues, promoting relaxation and reducing stress and anxiety.

Gua Sha

Gua Sha is a technique used in Tui Na application in Dit Da that involves the use of a tool to scrape the skin to promote blood flow and reduce pain and stiffness. The tool is usually made of stone, plastic, or metal and is scraped along the skin in a specific pattern.

Gua Sha can be particularly effective for treating musculoskeletal injuries and conditions, as well as respiratory conditions and digestive disorders. By promoting blood flow, Gua Sha can help to reduce pain and inflammation, improve circulation, and promote healing in the affected area.

Chapter Six

Qi Gong and Dit Da

Qi Gong is a traditional Chinese practice that involves the use of various physical and mental exercises to promote the flow of energy, or qi, in the body and improve overall health and well-being. In martial arts training, Qi Gong is often used in conjunction with Dit Da to aid in the treatment of musculoskeletal injuries and conditions.

Here are some facts about Qi Gong and how it relates to Dit Da.

History of Qi Gong

Qi Gong can be traced back to ancient China, where it was developed as a form of exercise and meditation to promote overall health and well-being. Over time, the practice evolved to include various physical exercises, including stretching, breathing techniques, and meditation.

Today, Qi Gong is practiced all over the world, with many practitioners using the techniques to promote healing and improve overall health and well-being.

The Meridian System and Qi Gong

One of the primary principles of Qi Gong is the concept of the meridian system and the flow of energy, or qi, through the body. In traditional Chinese medicine, it is believed that the body is composed of various channels, or meridians, through which qi flows.

Qi Gong is based on the principle that stimulating the flow of qi through the meridian system can promote healing and improve overall health and well-being. This principle is closely related to the practice of Dit Da, which also seeks to stimulate the flow of energy in the body to aid in the healing process.

Physical Exercises in Qi Gong

Qi Gong involves the use of various physical exercises to promote the flow of energy, or qi, in the body. These exercises can include stretching, breathing techniques, and meditation.

By promoting the flow of qi, Qi Gong can help to reduce stress and anxiety, improve circulation, and promote healing in the body. This principle is closely related to the practice of Dit Da, which also seeks to promote healing through the manipulation of soft tissues and stimulation of energy flow in the body.

Mental Exercises in Qi Gong

In addition to physical exercises, Qi Gong also involves the use of mental exercises, including visualization and meditation, to promote healing and improve overall health and well-being.

These exercises can be particularly effective for reducing stress and anxiety, promoting relaxation, and improving mental clarity. This principle is closely related to the practice of Dit Da, which also seeks to promote relaxation and reduce stress and anxiety through the use of massage and other therapeutic techniques.

Qi Gong and Dit Da

Qi Gong and Dit Da are closely related practices that share many similarities in their principles and techniques. Both practices seek to promote the flow of energy, or qi, in the body to aid in the healing process and improve overall health and well-being.

In martial arts training, Qi Gong is often used in conjunction with Dit Da to provide a comprehensive approach to healing and wellness. Together, these practices can help to reduce pain and inflammation, improve circulation, promote relaxation, and reduce stress and anxiety.

The role of Qi Gong in

Dit

Da therapy

Dit Da therapy is a traditional Chinese medicine practice that is often used in conjunction with martial arts training to aid in the treatment of musculoskeletal injuries and conditions. Qi Gong is another traditional Chinese practice that involves the use of various physical and mental exercises to promote the flow of energy, or qi, in the body and improve overall health and well-being.

Here are some facts about the role of Qi Gong in Dit Da therapy.

Stimulating Energy Flow

One of the primary principles of Qi Gong is the concept of energy flow, or qi. In traditional Chinese medicine, it is believed that the body is composed of various channels, or meridians, through which qi flows.

Qi Gong is based on the principle that stimulating the flow of qi through the meridian system can promote healing and improve overall health and well-being. This principle is closely related to the practice of Dit Da, which also seeks to stimulate the flow of energy in the body to aid in the healing process.

Reducing Stress and Anxiety

Qi Gong involves the use of various physical and mental exercises to reduce stress and anxiety, promote relaxation, and improve mental clarity. These exercises can be particularly effective for reducing stress and anxiety, promoting relaxation, and improving mental clarity. This principle is closely related to the practice of Dit Da, which also seeks to promote relaxation and reduce stress and anxiety through the use of massage and other therapeutic techniques.

Improving Circulation

Qi Gong can also help to improve circulation in the body, promoting the flow of oxygen and nutrients to the affected area. This can be particularly effective for promoting healing in musculoskeletal injuries and conditions.

The improved circulation can also help to reduce inflammation and promote overall health and well-being. This principle is closely related to the practice of Dit Da, which also seeks to promote healing through the manipulation of soft tissues and stimulation of energy flow in the body.

Complementing Dit Da Therapy

Qi Gong can be an effective complement to Dit Da therapy, providing a comprehensive approach to healing and wellness. By working together, these practices can help to reduce pain and inflammation, improve circulation, promote relaxation, and reduce stress and anxiety.

Qi Gong can be practiced alongside other traditional Chinese medicine practices, such as acupuncture and herbal medicine, to provide a comprehensive approach to healing and wellness.

Breathing and energy cultivation exercises

Dit Da is a traditional Chinese medicine practice that is often used in martial arts training to aid in the treatment of musculoskeletal injuries and conditions. In addition to massage and other therapeutic techniques, Dit Da also involves the use of breathing and energy cultivation exercises to promote healing and improve overall health and well-being.

Here are some facts about breathing and energy cultivation exercises in Dit Da.

The Role of Breathing

Breathing is an essential component of Dit Da therapy. Proper breathing techniques can help to promote relaxation, reduce stress and anxiety, and improve overall health and well-being.

One of the primary breathing techniques used in Dit Da is abdominal breathing, also known as diaphragmatic breathing. This technique involves breathing deeply into the abdomen, allowing the diaphragm to expand fully, and exhaling slowly and deeply.

Abdominal breathing can be particularly effective for reducing stress and anxiety, promoting relaxation, and improving circulation in the body. This principle is closely related to the practice of Dit Da, which also seeks to promote healing through the manipulation of soft tissues and stimulation of energy flow in the body.

The Role of Energy Cultivation

Energy cultivation is another essential component of Dit Da therapy. This involves the use of various exercises and techniques to promote the flow of energy, or qi, in the body and improve overall health and well-being.

One of the primary energy cultivation techniques used in Dit Da is qigong, which involves the use of various physical and mental exercises to promote the flow of energy in the body. Qigong can help to reduce stress and anxiety, improve circulation, and promote relaxation, making it an effective complement to other Dit Da therapy techniques.

Another energy cultivation technique used in Dit Da is the practice of meditation, which can help to reduce stress and anxiety, improve mental clarity, and promote overall health and well-being.

Breathing and Energy Cultivation in Practice

Breathing and energy cultivation exercises can be incorporated into a regular Dit Da therapy practice to promote healing and improve overall health and well-being.

One common technique used in Dit Da is to combine breathing and energy cultivation exercises with massage and other therapeutic techniques. By incorporating deep breathing and energy cultivation into the massage practice, Dit Da practitioners can promote relaxation, reduce stress and anxiety, and improve circulation in the body.

Another common technique used in Dit Da is to incorporate breathing and energy cultivation exercises into a regular martial arts training practice. By practicing these exercises regularly, martial artists can improve their overall health and well-being, as well as their martial arts performance.

Chapter Seven

Acupuncture and Dit Da

Dit Da is a traditional Chinese medicine practice that is often used in martial arts training to aid in the treatment of musculoskeletal injuries and conditions. Acupuncture is another traditional Chinese medicine practice that involves the insertion of thin needles into specific points on the body to promote healing and improve overall health and well-being.

Here are some facts about acupuncture and its relationship to Dit Da.

History of Acupuncture

Acupuncture can be traced back to ancient China, where it was developed as a form of medicine to promote overall health and well-being. Over time, the practice evolved to include the use of needles to stimulate specific points on the body to promote healing.

Today, acupuncture is practiced all over the world, with many practitioners using the technique to treat a wide range of conditions, including musculoskeletal injuries.

The Meridian System and Acupuncture

One of the primary principles of acupuncture is the concept of the meridian system and the flow of energy, or qi, through the body. In traditional Chinese medicine, it is believed that the body is composed of various channels, or meridians, through which qi flows.

Acupuncture is based on the principle that stimulating specific points on the body can promote the flow of qi through the meridian system, aiding in the healing process and improving overall health and well-being. This principle is closely related to the practice of Dit Da, which also seeks to stimulate the flow of energy in the body to aid in the healing process.

Acupuncture Techniques

Acupuncture involves the insertion of thin needles into specific points on the body to stimulate the flow of energy and promote healing. These needles are typically left in place for several minutes to promote the desired effect.

In addition to needles, acupuncture can also involve the use of other techniques, such as cupping, which involves the use of suction cups to promote blood flow and reduce inflammation in the affected area.

Acupuncture and Dit Da

Acupuncture and Dit Da are closely related practices that share many similarities in their principles and techniques. Both practices seek to promote the flow of energy, or qi, in the body to aid in the healing process and improve overall health and well-being.

In martial arts training, acupuncture is often used in conjunction with Dit Da to provide a comprehensive approach to healing and wellness. Together, these practices can help to reduce pain and inflammation, improve circulation, promote relaxation, and reduce stress and anxiety.

Combining acupuncture with

Dit

Da therapy

Dit Da therapy is a traditional Chinese medicine practice that is often used in martial arts training to aid in the treatment of musculoskeletal injuries and conditions. Acupuncture is another traditional Chinese medicine practice that involves the insertion of thin needles into specific points on the body to promote healing and improve overall health and well-being.

Here are some facts about the benefits of combining acupuncture with Dit Da therapy.

Improved Circulation

Acupuncture and Dit Da therapy can both help to improve circulation in the body, promoting the flow of oxygen and nutrients to the affected area. This can be particularly effective for promoting healing in musculoskeletal injuries and conditions.

By working together, acupuncture and Dit Da therapy can provide a comprehensive approach to improving circulation and promoting healing.

Reduced Inflammation

Both acupuncture and Dit Da therapy can help to reduce inflammation in the body. Acupuncture works by stimulating the release of anti-inflammatory compounds in the body, while Dit Da therapy works by manipulating the soft tissues to promote healing.

By combining these two practices, practitioners can provide a more comprehensive approach to reducing inflammation and promoting healing.

Stress and Anxiety Reduction

Acupuncture and Dit Da therapy can both help to reduce stress and anxiety, promoting relaxation and improving overall well-being. Acupuncture works by stimulating the release of endorphins, which are natural painkillers and mood boosters. Dit Da therapy works by manipulating the soft tissues to promote relaxation.

Together, these practices can provide a comprehensive approach to reducing stress and anxiety and improving overall well-being.

Improved Energy Flow

Acupuncture and Dit Da therapy both seek to improve the flow of energy, or qi, in the body. Acupuncture works by stimulating specific points on the body to promote the flow of energy, while Dit Da therapy works by manipulating the soft tissues to promote energy flow.

By combining these practices, practitioners can provide a more comprehensive approach to improving energy flow and promoting overall health and well-being.

Comprehensive Approach to Healing

By combining acupuncture and Dit Da therapy, practitioners can provide a more comprehensive approach to healing and wellness. Together, these practices can help to reduce pain and inflammation, improve circulation, promote relaxation, reduce stress and anxiety, and improve overall well-being.

Acupuncture and Dit Da therapy can also be combined with other traditional Chinese medicine practices, such as herbal medicine, to provide a more comprehensive approach to healing and wellness.

Meridians and acupoints related to

Dit

Da

Dit Da is a traditional Chinese medicine practice that is often used in martial arts training to aid in the treatment of musculoskeletal injuries and conditions. Central to this practice are the concepts of meridians and acupoints.

Here are some facts about meridians and acupoints related to Dit Da.

Meridians

In traditional Chinese medicine, meridians are the channels through which qi, or vital energy, flows throughout the body. These meridians are believed to correspond to specific organs and organ systems in the body and are often associated with specific physical and emotional functions.

There are 12 primary meridians in the body, each associated with a specific organ system. These meridians run in a network throughout the body, with each meridian having its own specific pathway.

Dit Da practitioners use the concept of meridians to identify the root cause of musculoskeletal injuries and conditions. By understanding which meridians are affected by an injury or condition, practitioners can develop targeted treatment plans to promote healing and reduce pain and inflammation.

Acupoints

Acupoints are specific points along the meridians where the flow of qi can be manipulated to promote healing and wellness. Acupoints are located throughout the body and are often associated with specific organs or organ systems.

In Dit Da practice, acupoints are used to manipulate the flow of energy in the body to promote healing and reduce pain and inflammation. Acupoints are typically stimulated using pressure, massage, or the insertion of needles.

There are hundreds of acupoints throughout the body, each with its own specific function and location. In Dit Da practice, acupoints are often targeted based on the location and severity of the injury or condition.

Common Acupoints Related to Dit Da

Here are some common acupoints related to Dit Da and their associated functions:

Large Intestine 4 (LI 4) - This acupoint is located on the hand, between the thumb and index finger. It is often used to relieve pain and reduce inflammation in the upper body.

Gallbladder 34 (GB 34) - This acupoint is located on the foot, near the ankle. It is often used to relieve pain and reduce inflammation in the lower body.

Stomach 36 (ST 36) - This acupoint is located on the lower leg, below the knee. It is often used to improve circulation and promote overall well-being.

Pericardium 6 (PC 6) - This acupoint is located on the inside of the wrist. It is often used to relieve stress and anxiety and promote relaxation.

Bladder 40 (BL 40) - This acupoint is located on the back of the leg, behind the knee. It is often used to relieve pain and reduce inflammation in the lower body.

Chapter Eight

Cupping Therapy in Dit Da

Cupping therapy is a traditional Chinese medicine practice that involves the use of cups to create suction on the skin. This practice has been used for centuries to promote healing, improve circulation, and reduce pain and inflammation. In Dit Da practice, cupping therapy is often used as a complementary therapy to aid in the treatment of musculoskeletal injuries and conditions.

Here are some facts about cupping therapy in Dit Da.

History of Cupping Therapy

Cupping therapy has been used in traditional Chinese medicine for over 2,000 years. Originally, cups were made from animal horns and were used to draw out toxins from the body. Later, cups were made from bamboo, ceramic, or glass and were used to treat a variety of conditions, including musculoskeletal injuries and conditions.

Today, cupping therapy is still used in traditional Chinese medicine and is gaining popularity in the Western world as well.

How Cupping Therapy Works

Cupping therapy works by creating suction on the skin, which can help to improve circulation, reduce pain and inflammation, and promote healing.

During a cupping therapy session, cups are placed on the skin and a vacuum is created either by heating the air inside the cup or by using a pump. The cups are left in place for a few minutes, creating suction on the skin.

Cupping therapy can be performed on different parts of the body, depending on the condition being treated. In Dit Da practice, cupping therapy is often used on the back, shoulders, and other areas of the body affected by musculoskeletal injuries and conditions.

Benefits of Cupping Therapy in Dit Da

Cupping therapy can provide a range of benefits in Dit Da practice, including:

Improved circulation - Cupping therapy can help to improve circulation in the affected area, promoting the flow of oxygen and nutrients to the injured tissues.

Reduced pain and inflammation - Cupping therapy can help to reduce pain and inflammation in the affected area, promoting healing and reducing discomfort.

Improved range of motion - Cupping therapy can help to improve range of motion in the affected area, allowing for a more comprehensive approach to healing.

Improved overall well-being - Cupping therapy can promote relaxation and improve overall well-being, reducing stress and anxiety.

Types of Cupping Therapy

There are several different types of cupping therapy used in traditional Chinese medicine, including:

Dry cupping - This is the most common type of cupping therapy, which involves creating suction on the skin using cups.

Wet cupping - This involves creating small incisions on the skin before applying the cups, allowing for the release of blood and toxins from the body.

Fire cupping - This involves heating the air inside the cups before applying them to the skin, creating suction.

In Dit Da practice, dry cupping is the most commonly used type of cupping therapy.

Precautions for Cupping Therapy

While cupping therapy is generally safe, there are some precautions that should be taken, particularly if you have certain medical conditions. These include:

Pregnant women should avoid cupping therapy on their lower back and abdomen.

People with bleeding disorders should avoid cupping therapy.

People with skin conditions or sensitivities may experience irritation from cupping therapy.

The benefits of cupping for

Dit

Da

Cupping therapy is a traditional Chinese medicine practice that has been used for centuries to promote healing, improve circulation, and reduce pain and inflammation. In Dit Da practice, cupping therapy is often used as a complementary therapy to aid in the treatment of musculoskeletal injuries and conditions. Here are some of the benefits of cupping therapy for Dit Da.

Promotes Blood Flow

Cupping therapy can promote blood flow in the affected area, which can help to reduce pain and inflammation and promote healing. The suction created by the cups can help to draw blood to the area, providing the necessary nutrients and oxygen to promote healing.

Reduces Pain and Inflammation

Cupping therapy can help to reduce pain and inflammation in the affected area. The suction created by the cups can help to release tension and promote relaxation, which can help to reduce pain and discomfort.

Improves Range of Motion

Cupping therapy can help to improve range of motion in the affected area. The suction created by the cups can help to release tension and tightness in the muscles, allowing for greater flexibility and movement.

Enhances Overall Well-being

Cupping therapy can enhance overall well-being by promoting relaxation and reducing stress and anxiety. This can have a positive impact on the body's ability to heal and recover from injuries and conditions.

Reduces Scar Tissue

Cupping therapy can help to reduce scar tissue in the affected area. The suction created by the cups can help to break up scar tissue, promoting healing and reducing discomfort.

Increases Immune Function

Cupping therapy can increase immune function in the body, which can help to promote healing and reduce the risk of infections. By promoting blood flow and reducing inflammation, cupping therapy can help the body's natural immune response to function more efficiently.

Types of Cupping Therapy

There are several different types of cupping therapy used in traditional Chinese medicine, including:

Dry cupping - This is the most common type of cupping therapy, which involves creating suction on the skin using cups.

Wet cupping - This involves creating small incisions on the skin before applying the cups, allowing for the release of blood and toxins from the body.

Fire cupping - This involves heating the air inside the cups before applying them to the skin, creating suction.

In Dit Da practice, dry cupping is the most commonly used type of cupping therapy.

Precautions for Cupping Therapy

While cupping therapy is generally safe, there are some precautions that should be taken, particularly if you have certain medical conditions. These include:

Pregnant women should avoid cupping therapy on their lower back and abdomen.

People with bleeding disorders should avoid cupping therapy.

People with skin conditions or sensitivities may experience irritation from cupping therapy.

Techniques and safety precautions

Dit Da is a traditional Chinese medicine practice that involves the use of different techniques to treat musculoskeletal injuries and conditions. While it can be an effective treatment option, it is important to take proper safety precautions to ensure the well-being of both the practitioner and the patient. Here are some techniques and safety precautions to consider in Dit Da practice.

Techniques

Massage - Massage is a common technique used in Dit Da practice to promote healing and reduce pain and inflammation. Different massage techniques can be used depending on the injury or condition being treated.

Acupuncture - Acupuncture is a technique used in Dit Da practice to help promote healing and reduce pain and inflammation. Thin needles are inserted into specific points in the body to help restore balance and promote healing.

Cupping - Cupping therapy involves creating suction on the skin to promote blood flow, reduce pain and inflammation, and promote healing. Cups can be placed on different areas of the body depending on the injury or condition being treated.

Tui Na - Tui Na is a type of massage that involves pressing and kneading different points on the body to promote healing and reduce pain and inflammation.

Qi Gong - Qi Gong is a type of exercise that involves breathing techniques, meditation, and movement to promote overall well-being and reduce stress and anxiety.

Safety Precautions

Proper training - It is important for practitioners to receive proper training and certification in Dit Da practice to ensure they are using proper techniques and safety precautions.

Hygiene - Practitioners should ensure proper hygiene practices are followed, including washing hands before and after treatment, and using clean and sterilized equipment.

Patient assessment - Before beginning any treatment, practitioners should assess the patient's medical history, current condition, and any contraindications to ensure that the treatment is safe and effective.

Communication - Practitioners should communicate with their patients to ensure they understand the treatment plan and any potential risks or side effects.

Pain management - Pain management should be a top priority in Dit Da practice. Practitioners should ensure that patients are comfortable throughout the treatment and that pain is managed appropriately.

Personal protective equipment - Practitioners should wear personal protective equipment, such as gloves and masks, to reduce the risk of infection and protect themselves and their patients.

Chapter Nine

Gua Sha and Dit Da

Gua Sha is a traditional Chinese medicine practice that involves the use of a smooth tool, such as a jade or horn scraper, to scrape the skin and promote blood flow and healing. It has been used for centuries in Chinese medicine to treat a variety of conditions, including musculoskeletal injuries and pain. In Dit Da practice, Gua Sha is often used as a complementary therapy to aid in the treatment of injuries and conditions. Here are some important aspects of Gua Sha in relation to Dit Da.

Technique

Gua Sha involves the use of a smooth tool to apply pressure and scrape the skin in a particular pattern. The tool is usually applied to the affected area after applying oil or lotion to reduce friction. The practitioner applies pressure and moves the tool in a scraping motion along the skin, creating redness or bruising. The technique can be adjusted depending on the injury or condition being treated, and the pressure should be adjusted to the patient's comfort level.

Benefits

Gua Sha can provide a range of benefits for Dit Da practice, including promoting blood flow, reducing pain and inflammation, improving range of motion, and reducing muscle tension. The technique can also help to release toxins from the body and promote overall well-being.

Safety Precautions

While Gua Sha is generally considered safe, there are some precautions that should be taken to ensure the well-being of both the practitioner and the patient. These include:

Proper training - Practitioners should receive proper training in Gua Sha techniques and safety precautions to ensure that they are using the proper technique and avoiding any potential risks.

Hygiene - Practitioners should ensure proper hygiene practices are followed, including washing hands before and after treatment, and using clean and sterilized equipment.

Patient assessment - Before beginning any treatment, practitioners should assess the patient's medical history, current condition, and any contraindications to ensure that the treatment is safe and effective.

Communication - Practitioners should communicate with their patients to ensure they understand the treatment plan and any potential risks or side effects.

Pain management - Pain management should be a top priority in Gua Sha practice. Practitioners should ensure that patients are comfortable throughout the treatment and that pain is managed appropriately.

Avoiding bony areas - The practitioner should avoid scraping over bony areas or areas with delicate skin, such as the face or neck, to avoid injury.

Integrating Gua Sha into

Dit

Da practice

Dit Da is a traditional Chinese medicine practice that focuses on treating musculoskeletal injuries and conditions. Gua Sha is another traditional Chinese medicine practice that involves using a smooth tool to scrape the skin and promote blood flow and healing. When used together, Gua Sha can be a valuable addition to a comprehensive Dit Da practice. Here are some important aspects of integrating Gua Sha into Dit Da practice.

Benefits

Gua Sha can provide a range of benefits when integrated into Dit Da practice. It can promote blood flow to the affected area, reduce pain and inflammation, and help to release toxins from the body. By promoting healing and reducing pain and inflammation, Gua Sha can complement the other techniques used in Dit Da practice, such as massage, acupuncture, and cupping therapy.

Technique

Gua Sha is a technique that involves the use of a smooth tool, such as a jade or horn scraper, to scrape the skin in a particular pattern. The tool is usually applied to the affected area after applying oil or lotion to reduce friction. The practitioner applies pressure and moves the tool in a scraping motion along the skin, creating redness or bruising. The technique can be adjusted depending on the injury or condition being treated, and the pressure should be adjusted to the patient's comfort level.

Integrating Gua Sha into Dit Da Practice

Integrating Gua Sha into Dit Da practice involves incorporating the technique into the overall treatment plan for a patient. Here are some important considerations for integrating Gua Sha into Dit Da practice:

Patient Assessment - Before integrating Gua Sha into a patient's treatment plan, the practitioner should assess the patient's medical history, current condition, and any contraindications to ensure that the treatment is safe and effective.

Treatment Plan - Gua Sha should be integrated into the overall treatment plan for a patient, which may include other techniques such as massage, acupuncture, and cupping therapy. The treatment plan should be customized to the patient's specific injury or condition.

Technique - The Gua Sha technique should be adjusted based on the injury or condition being treated, and the pressure should be adjusted to the patient's comfort level. The practitioner should also ensure that they are using the proper technique to avoid any potential risks.

Communication - The practitioner should communicate with their patient to ensure they understand the treatment plan and any potential risks or side effects.

Pain Management - Pain management should be a top priority in Gua Sha practice. Practitioners should ensure that patients are comfortable throughout the treatment and that pain is managed appropriately.

Proper techniques and tools

Dit Da is a traditional Chinese medicine practice that focuses on treating musculoskeletal injuries and conditions. It uses a combination of techniques, including massage, acupuncture, cupping therapy, and herbal remedies, to promote healing and reduce pain. Proper techniques and tools are essential in Dit Da practice to ensure safe and effective treatment. Here are some important considerations for using proper techniques and tools in Dit Da practice.

Massage Techniques

Massage is a key technique in Dit Da practice and involves applying pressure to the affected area to promote healing and reduce pain. There are several massage techniques used in Dit Da practice, including:

Shiatsu - This technique involves applying pressure to specific points on the body using fingers, thumbs, or palms.

Tui Na - This technique involves kneading, rolling, and pressing the affected area using a variety of techniques.

An Mo - This technique involves kneading and rubbing the affected area to promote blood flow and reduce pain.

Gua Sha - This technique involves using a smooth tool to scrape the skin and promote blood flow and healing.

Proper techniques are essential to ensure that massage is safe and effective. The practitioner should adjust the technique based on the patient's injury or condition, and the pressure should be adjusted to the patient's comfort level.

Acupuncture Techniques

Acupuncture is another key technique in Dit Da practice and involves inserting thin needles into specific points on the body to promote healing and reduce pain. Proper techniques are essential to ensure that acupuncture is safe and effective. The practitioner should use sterile needles and insert them at the proper depth and angle based on the patient's injury or condition.

Cupping Therapy Techniques

Cupping therapy is another technique used in Dit Da practice and involves placing cups on the skin to create suction and promote blood flow and healing. Proper techniques are essential to ensure that cupping therapy is safe and effective. The practitioner should adjust the amount of suction based on the patient's comfort level and adjust the placement of the cups based on the patient's injury or condition.

Herbal Remedies

Herbal remedies are often used in Dit Da practice to promote healing and reduce pain. Proper techniques are essential to ensure that herbal remedies are safe and effective. The practitioner should use high-quality herbs and adjust the dosage based on the patient's injury or condition.

Tools

Proper tools are essential in Dit Da practice to ensure safe and effective treatment. Here are some important considerations for using proper tools in Dit Da practice:

Sterilization - All tools should be sterilized before use to prevent the spread of infection.

Quality - High-quality tools should be used to ensure that they are durable and effective.

Safety - All tools should be used in a safe manner to prevent injury to the patient.

Adjustability - Some tools, such as massage tools, should be adjustable to ensure that they can be used on different parts of the body and adjusted based on the patient's injury or condition.

Chapter Ten

Moxibustion and Dit Da

Moxibustion is a traditional Chinese medicine practice that involves burning an herb called moxa (Artemisia vulgaris) to promote healing and reduce pain. It is commonly used in conjunction with acupuncture and massage in Dit Da practice to treat musculoskeletal injuries and conditions. Below we will explore the history of moxibustion, how it works, and its role in Dit Da practice.

History of Moxibustion

Moxibustion has a long history in traditional Chinese medicine and is believed to have originated in ancient China over 2,500 years ago. The practice involves burning dried moxa on specific points on the body to stimulate circulation and promote healing. The use of moxa was first recorded in the Huangdi Neijing (The Yellow Emperor's Classic of Internal Medicine), which is one of the oldest and most important texts in traditional Chinese medicine.

How Moxibustion Works

Moxibustion is based on the principles of traditional Chinese medicine, which views the body as a complex system of interconnected meridians or pathways through which energy, or qi, flows. According to this theory, health is achieved when the flow of qi is balanced and unobstructed, while illness and pain result from imbalances or blockages in the flow of qi.

Moxibustion works by stimulating the flow of qi and promoting healing. When moxa is burned on specific points on the body, the heat and smoke produced by the burning herb stimulate the flow of qi and increase circulation. This helps to promote healing and reduce pain.

Types of Moxibustion

There are several types of moxibustion used in traditional Chinese medicine, including:

Direct moxibustion - This involves placing a small amount of moxa directly on the skin and burning it until it is extinguished.

Indirect moxibustion - This involves using a moxa stick, which is a stick made of compressed moxa, to warm the skin without burning it.

Heat lamp moxibustion - This involves using a heat lamp to warm the skin and promote healing.

Smokeless moxibustion - This involves using a moxa stick that produces minimal smoke to avoid the inhalation of harmful chemicals.

Role of Moxibustion in Dit Da Practice

Moxibustion is commonly used in Dit Da practice to treat musculoskeletal injuries and conditions. It is often used in conjunction with acupuncture and massage to promote healing and reduce pain. Moxibustion is believed to be especially effective for treating conditions that are related to cold and dampness, such as arthritis and joint pain.

Moxibustion is also believed to be effective for promoting overall health and well-being. Regular moxibustion treatments are believed to help boost the immune system, increase energy, and reduce stress and anxiety.

Safety Considerations

While moxibustion is generally safe when performed by a trained practitioner, there are some safety considerations to keep in mind. The burning moxa can produce smoke and ash, which can be inhaled and cause respiratory problems. For this reason, it is important to use smokeless moxa or to perform moxibustion in a well-ventilated area.

Moxibustion should also not be used on pregnant women or people with certain medical conditions, such as epilepsy or skin conditions. It is important to consult with a trained practitioner before undergoing moxibustion treatment.

The role of moxibustion in

Dit

Da healing

Dit Da is a traditional Chinese medicine practice that focuses on the prevention and treatment of musculoskeletal injuries and conditions. It encompasses various techniques, including massage, acupuncture, bone setting, and herbal medicine. Moxibustion is another technique that is commonly used in Dit Da practice to promote healing and reduce pain. Below we will explore the role of moxibustion in Dit Da healing.

What is Moxibustion?

Moxibustion is a traditional Chinese medicine practice that involves burning an herb called moxa (Artemisia vulgaris) to stimulate circulation and promote healing. Moxa is usually made from the dried leaves of the mugwort plant and is often used in conjunction with acupuncture, massage, and other traditional Chinese medicine techniques.

How Does Moxibustion Work?

Moxibustion works by stimulating the flow of Qi, the vital energy that is believed to flow through the body's meridians or energy pathways. According to traditional Chinese medicine, when Qi is flowing smoothly, the body is healthy, and when it is blocked or stagnant, illness and pain can result.

During a moxibustion treatment, the practitioner places a small amount of moxa on a specific point on the body and burns it. The heat and smoke produced by the burning moxa penetrate deep into the tissues and stimulate the flow of Qi, promoting healing and reducing pain.

The Role of Moxibustion in Dit Da Healing

Moxibustion is a valuable technique in Dit Da practice because it can be used to treat a wide range of musculoskeletal injuries and conditions. Some of the common conditions that can be treated with moxibustion include:

1. Arthritis and Joint Pain: Moxibustion is often used to treat joint pain and stiffness caused by arthritis. The heat produced by the burning moxa helps to reduce inflammation and promote blood flow to the affected area, reducing pain and improving mobility.

2. Muscle Strains and Sprains: Moxibustion can also be used to treat muscle strains and sprains. The heat and smoke produced by the burning moxa penetrate deep into the tissues, helping to reduce inflammation and promote healing.

3. Back Pain: Moxibustion is a common treatment for back pain. The heat produced by the burning moxa can help to relax the muscles and reduce tension, relieving pain and stiffness in the back.

4. Digestive Disorders: Moxibustion can also be used to treat digestive disorders, such as irritable bowel syndrome (IBS) and indigestion. The heat produced by the burning moxa can help to stimulate digestion and reduce inflammation in the digestive tract.

5. Respiratory Disorders: Moxibustion can be used to treat respiratory disorders, such as asthma and bronchitis. The heat and smoke produced by the burning moxa can help to open up the airways and reduce inflammation in the lungs.

Proper Techniques and Safety Precautions

Moxibustion should always be performed by a trained practitioner who has experience in traditional Chinese medicine. The practitioner will choose the appropriate points on the body to stimulate and the correct type of moxibustion to use.

It is important to follow safety precautions when undergoing moxibustion treatment. The burning moxa can produce smoke and ash, which can be inhaled and cause respiratory problems. For this reason, it is important to use smokeless moxa or to perform moxibustion in a well-ventilated area.

Moxibustion should not be used on pregnant women or people with certain medical conditions, such as epilepsy or skin conditions. It is important to consult with a trained practitioner before undergoing moxibustion treatment

Techniques for using moxa in

Dit

Da therapy

Dit Da therapy is a traditional Chinese medicine practice that focuses on the prevention and treatment of musculoskeletal injuries and conditions. One of the techniques used in Dit Da therapy is moxibustion, which involves burning an herb called moxa (Artemisia vulgaris) to promote healing and reduce pain. Below we will explore the various techniques for using moxa in Dit Da therapy.

Direct Moxibustion

Direct moxibustion is a technique where the practitioner places a small amount of moxa directly on the skin at the acupoint or area of injury. The moxa is lit and allowed to burn for a few minutes until the skin becomes red and warm.

Direct moxibustion can be used to treat a wide range of musculoskeletal injuries, including muscle strains, sprains, and joint pain. The heat produced by the burning moxa penetrates deep into the tissues, promoting blood flow and reducing pain and inflammation.

Indirect Moxibustion

Indirect moxibustion is a technique where the practitioner holds a burning moxa stick close to the skin without actually touching it. The heat produced by the burning moxa is transferred to the skin, promoting healing and reducing pain.

Indirect moxibustion is a gentler technique than direct moxibustion and is often used to treat more delicate areas of the body, such as the face or neck. It can also be used to treat conditions such as digestive disorders, respiratory problems, and menstrual cramps.

Cupping Moxibustion

Cupping moxibustion is a technique where a small amount of moxa is placed on an acupoint, and then a cup is placed over the moxa to create a vacuum. The heat produced by the burning moxa penetrates deep into the tissues, promoting blood flow and reducing pain and inflammation.

Cupping moxibustion is often used to treat conditions such as back pain, menstrual cramps, and respiratory disorders. The vacuum created by the cupping technique helps to improve blood flow and lymphatic drainage, promoting healing and reducing pain.

Moxa Rollers

Moxa rollers are another technique used in Dit Da therapy. The practitioner rolls a moxa stick over the skin at the acupoint or area of injury, applying heat and pressure to promote healing and reduce pain.

Moxa rollers can be used to treat a wide range of musculoskeletal injuries, including muscle strains, sprains, and joint pain. The heat and pressure produced by the moxa roller penetrate deep into the tissues, promoting blood flow and reducing pain and inflammation.

Moxa Cones

Moxa cones are a small cone-shaped moxa stick that is used to stimulate the acupoints. The cone is placed on top of the acupoint and lit, producing heat that penetrates deep into the tissues.

Moxa cones can be used to treat a wide range of musculoskeletal injuries, including back pain, neck pain, and joint pain. The heat produced by the burning moxa helps to reduce pain and inflammation and promote healing.

Safety Precautions

Moxibustion is generally safe when performed by a trained practitioner. However, there are some safety precautions that should be followed to ensure that the treatment is safe and effective.

First, it is important to use high-quality moxa that is free from impurities and contaminants. The moxa should also be stored properly to prevent it from becoming damp or moldy.

Second, it is important to use moxibustion only under the supervision of a trained practitioner. The practitioner will choose the appropriate points on the body to stimulate and the correct type of moxibustion to use.

Chapter Eleven

Herbal Plasters and Liniments

Herbal plasters and liniments are traditional Chinese medicine techniques used in Dit Da therapy to treat musculoskeletal injuries and conditions. These topical treatments are made from a combination of herbs that are ground into a powder and mixed with a binding agent such as rice flour or honey.

Herbal plasters and liniments are applied directly to the skin at the site of the injury or to acupoints along the meridians. They are believed to work by promoting blood flow and reducing inflammation, helping to speed up the healing process.

Herbal Plasters

Herbal plasters are made by mixing ground herbs with a binding agent and water to create a paste. The paste is then spread onto a piece of gauze or cloth and applied to the skin.

Herbal plasters are often used to treat chronic or long-term injuries, such as arthritis or tendonitis. The herbs in the plaster penetrate deep into the tissues, providing sustained relief from pain and inflammation.

Some common herbs used in herbal plasters include:

1. Arnica: Arnica is a plant that is often used to treat bruises, sprains, and strains. It is believed to reduce inflammation and pain.

2. Frankincense: Frankincense is a resin that is often used to treat joint pain and inflammation. It is believed to have anti-inflammatory and analgesic properties.

3. Myrrh: Myrrh is a resin that is often used to treat muscle pain and inflammation. It is believed to have antispasmodic and analgesic properties.

Herbal Liniments

Herbal liniments are made by steeping herbs in alcohol or vinegar to extract their active ingredients. The resulting liquid is then applied to the skin using a cloth or cotton ball.

Herbal liniments are often used to treat acute injuries, such as sprains or strains. The alcohol or vinegar helps to penetrate the skin, delivering the active ingredients directly to the affected area.

Some common herbs used in herbal liniments include:

4. Ginger: Ginger is often used to treat muscle pain and inflammation. It is believed to have anti-inflammatory and analgesic properties.

5. Turmeric: Turmeric is often used to treat joint pain and inflammation. It is believed to have anti-inflammatory and antioxidant properties.

6. Eucalyptus: Eucalyptus is often used to treat respiratory problems, such as asthma or bronchitis. It is believed to have anti-inflammatory and antimicrobial properties.

Safety Precautions

While herbal plasters and liniments are generally safe when used as directed, there are some precautions that should be taken to ensure that they are used safely and effectively.

First, it is important to choose high-quality herbs that are free from contaminants and impurities. The herbs should be sourced from a reputable supplier and stored properly to prevent spoilage.

Second, it is important to follow the instructions provided by the practitioner or on the packaging carefully. The amount of plaster or liniment to use and the frequency of application may vary depending on the individual and the injury being treated.

Finally, it is important to watch for any adverse reactions, such as itching or redness, and to stop using the plaster or liniment if these occur. If you have any concerns about using herbal plasters or liniments, talk to your healthcare provider or a trained practitioner in traditional Chinese medicine.

The use of topical remedies in

Dit

Da

Dit Da, also known as "hit medicine," is a traditional Chinese therapy used to treat injuries caused by trauma, such as bruises, sprains, and fractures. Topical remedies are often used in Dit Da therapy to help relieve pain, reduce inflammation, and promote healing.

Topical remedies may include herbal plasters, liniments, oils, and poultices. These remedies are applied directly to the skin at the site of the injury or to acupoints along the meridians to help stimulate circulation and promote healing.

Herbal Plasters

Herbal plasters are made by grinding herbs into a fine powder and mixing them with a binding agent, such as honey or rice flour. The mixture is then applied to a piece of gauze or cloth and placed directly on the skin.

The herbs used in herbal plasters vary depending on the injury being treated. For example, arnica is often used to treat bruises, while frankincense and myrrh are often used to treat joint pain and inflammation.

Herbal Liniments

Herbal liniments are made by steeping herbs in alcohol or vinegar to extract their active ingredients. The resulting liquid is then applied to the skin using a cloth or cotton ball.

Herbal liniments are often used to treat acute injuries, such as sprains and strains. Ginger, turmeric, and eucalyptus are common herbs used in herbal liniments due to their anti-inflammatory and analgesic properties.

Herbal Oils

Herbal oils are made by steeping herbs in a carrier oil, such as sesame or coconut oil, for several weeks. The resulting oil is then strained and used topically to help reduce pain and inflammation.

Herbal oils are often used to treat chronic conditions, such as arthritis and tendonitis. Common herbs used in herbal oils include cayenne pepper, ginger, and lavender.

Herbal Poultices

Herbal poultices are made by mashing fresh herbs into a paste and applying the mixture directly to the skin. The poultice is then covered with a cloth or bandage and left in place for several hours.

Herbal poultices are often used to treat acute injuries, such as bruises and sprains. Common herbs used in herbal poultices include comfrey, arnica, and chamomile.

Safety Precautions

While topical remedies are generally safe when used as directed, there are some precautions that should be taken to ensure their safety and effectiveness.

First, it is important to choose high-quality herbs that are free from contaminants and impurities. The herbs should be sourced from a reputable supplier and stored properly to prevent spoilage.

Second, it is important to follow the instructions provided by the practitioner or on the packaging carefully. The amount of remedy to use and the frequency of application may vary depending on the individual and the injury being treated.

Finally, it is important to watch for any adverse reactions, such as itching or redness, and to stop using the remedy if these occur. If you have any concerns about using topical remedies, talk to your healthcare provider or a trained practitioner in traditional Chinese medicine.

Common recipes and ingredients

Dit Da is a traditional Chinese therapy used to treat injuries caused by trauma, such as bruises, sprains, and fractures. In Dit Da therapy, various herbal remedies are used to help promote healing and relieve pain. These remedies may be applied topically, taken internally as teas or tinctures, or used in the form of pills or powders. Below we will discuss some common recipes and ingredients used in Dit Da therapy.

Arnica

Arnica is a perennial herb that is native to Europe and North America. The dried flowers of the arnica plant are used in Dit Da therapy to treat bruises, sprains, and muscle pain. Arnica contains compounds that help reduce inflammation and relieve pain.

To use arnica in Dit Da therapy, the dried flowers can be made into a poultice or a liniment. To make a poultice, mix the dried flowers with water to make a paste and apply it to the affected area. To make a liniment, steep the dried flowers in alcohol or vinegar for several weeks and then apply the resulting liquid to the skin.

Comfrey

Comfrey is a perennial herb that is native to Europe and Asia. The root and leaves of the comfrey plant are used in Dit Da therapy to treat bruises, sprains, and fractures. Comfrey contains compounds that help reduce inflammation and promote healing.

To use comfrey in Dit Da therapy, the leaves or root can be made into a poultice or a liniment. To make a poultice, mash the leaves or root into a paste and apply it to the affected area. To make a liniment, steep the leaves or root in alcohol or vinegar for several weeks and then apply the resulting liquid to the skin.

Ginger

Ginger is a root that is native to Asia. The root of the ginger plant is used in Dit Da therapy to treat joint pain and inflammation. Ginger contains compounds that help reduce inflammation and relieve pain.

To use ginger in Dit Da therapy, the root can be made into a poultice or a liniment. To make a poultice, grate the ginger root and mix it with water to make a paste. Apply the paste to the affected area and cover with a cloth or bandage. To make a liniment, steep the grated ginger root in alcohol or vinegar for several weeks and then apply the resulting liquid to the skin.

Angelica

Angelica is a perennial herb that is native to Europe and Asia. The root of the angelica plant is used in Dit Da therapy to treat bruises and joint pain. Angelica contains compounds that help promote blood circulation and relieve pain.

To use angelica in Dit Da therapy, the root can be made into a poultice or a liniment. To make a poultice, mash the root into a paste and apply it to the affected area. To make a liniment, steep the root in alcohol or vinegar for several weeks and then apply the resulting liquid to the skin.

Moxa

Moxa is a dried herb that is made from the leaves of the mugwort plant. Moxa is used in Dit Da therapy to promote healing and relieve pain. Moxa contains compounds that help promote blood circulation and relieve pain.

To use moxa in Dit Da therapy, the dried herb can be burned and applied to the skin. The heat from the burning moxa helps to stimulate blood flow and promote healing. Moxa can also be used in the form of a stick, which is held close to the skin to provide heat therapy.

Chapter Twelve

Healing Bruises and Contusions

Bruises and contusions are common injuries that can be caused by trauma, such as a fall, collision, or impact. These injuries can cause pain, swelling, and discoloration of the skin. In traditional Chinese medicine, Dit Da therapy is often used to treat bruises and contusions. Below we will discuss some techniques used in Dit Da therapy for healing bruises and contusions.

Ice Therapy

One of the most effective ways to reduce pain and swelling from a bruise or contusion is to apply ice to the affected area. Ice therapy helps to constrict blood vessels and reduce blood flow to the injured area, which can help to reduce inflammation and pain.

To use ice therapy for a bruise or contusion, wrap ice or a cold pack in a towel and apply it to the affected area for 15-20 minutes at a time, several times a day. It is important not to apply ice directly to the skin, as this can cause frostbite.

Herbal Plasters and Liniments

Herbal plasters and liniments are often used in Dit Da therapy to help promote healing and reduce pain and inflammation in bruises and contusions. These remedies may contain a variety of herbs, such as arnica, comfrey, and angelica, that have anti-inflammatory and pain-relieving properties.

To use an herbal plaster, mix the herbs with water to make a paste and apply it to the affected area. Cover the area with a cloth or bandage and leave it on for several hours, or overnight. To use an herbal liniment, steep the herbs in alcohol or vinegar for several weeks and then apply the resulting liquid to the skin.

Massage Therapy

Massage therapy can be a useful technique for promoting blood flow and reducing pain and inflammation in bruises and contusions. Massage helps to stimulate circulation and lymphatic flow, which can help to reduce swelling and promote healing.

To perform massage therapy for a bruise or contusion, use gentle, circular motions with the fingertips or palm of the hand to massage the area around the injury. Start with light pressure and gradually increase pressure as the area becomes less tender. It is important not to apply too much pressure, as this can cause further injury to the affected area.

Acupuncture

Acupuncture is a traditional Chinese therapy that involves inserting thin needles into specific points on the body. Acupuncture is often used in Dit Da therapy to help reduce pain and inflammation in bruises and contusions.

To use acupuncture for a bruise or contusion, the therapist will insert needles into specific acupoints around the injured area. These acupoints are believed to help stimulate circulation and promote healing in the affected area. Acupuncture is generally considered safe when performed by a trained practitioner.

Moxibustion

Moxibustion is a therapy that involves burning dried mugwort over specific acupoints on the body. Moxibustion is often used in Dit Da therapy to help promote blood flow and reduce pain and inflammation in bruises and contusions.

To use moxibustion for a bruise or contusion, the therapist will burn a small amount of dried mugwort over specific acupoints around the injured area. The heat from the burning moxa helps to stimulate circulation and promote healing in the affected area.

Strategies for treating bruises

Bruises are a common injury that occur when small blood vessels under the skin are damaged, causing blood to leak into the surrounding tissues. This can cause pain, tenderness, and discoloration of the skin. While most bruises will heal on their own within a few weeks, there are several strategies that can be used to help speed up the healing process and reduce pain and inflammation. In traditional Chinese medicine, Dit Da therapy is often used to treat bruises. Below we will discuss some strategies for treating bruises using Dit Da therapy.

Ice Therapy

Ice therapy is a simple and effective way to reduce pain and swelling from a bruise. Applying ice to the affected area helps to constrict blood vessels and reduce blood flow to the injured area, which can help to reduce inflammation and pain. To use ice therapy, wrap ice or a cold pack in a towel and apply it to the affected area for 15-20 minutes at a time, several times a day. It is important not to apply ice directly to the skin, as this can cause frostbite.

Herbal Plasters and Liniments

Herbal plasters and liniments are often used in Dit Da therapy to help promote healing and reduce pain and inflammation in bruises. These remedies may contain a variety of herbs, such as arnica, comfrey, and angelica, that have anti-inflammatory and pain-relieving properties. To use an herbal plaster, mix the herbs with water to make a paste and apply it to the affected area. Cover the area with a cloth or bandage and leave it on for several hours, or overnight. To use an herbal liniment, steep the herbs in alcohol or vinegar for several weeks and then apply the resulting liquid to the skin.

Massage Therapy

Massage therapy can be a useful technique for promoting blood flow and reducing pain and inflammation in bruises. Massage helps to stimulate circulation and lymphatic flow, which can help to reduce swelling and promote healing. To perform massage therapy for a bruise, use gentle, circular motions with the fingertips or palm of the hand to massage the area around the injury. Start with light pressure and gradually increase pressure as the area becomes less tender. It is important not to apply too much pressure, as this can cause further injury to the affected area.

Acupuncture

Acupuncture is a traditional Chinese therapy that involves inserting thin needles into specific points on the body. Acupuncture is often used in Dit Da therapy to help reduce pain and inflammation in bruises. To use acupuncture for a bruise, the therapist will insert needles into specific acupoints around the injured area. These acupoints are believed to help stimulate circulation and promote healing in the affected area. Acupuncture is generally considered safe when performed by a trained practitioner.

Moxibustion

Moxibustion is a therapy that involves burning dried mugwort over specific acupoints on the body. Moxibustion is often used in Dit Da therapy to help promote blood flow and reduce pain and inflammation in bruises. To use moxibustion for a bruise, the therapist will burn a small amount of dried mugwort over specific acupoints around the injured area. The heat from the burning moxa helps to stimulate circulation and promote healing in the affected area.

Herbal Teas

Herbal teas can be a useful strategy for reducing pain and inflammation from bruises. Chamomile tea, for example, has anti-inflammatory properties that can help to reduce swelling and pain. Ginger tea is another useful option, as it has natural pain-relieving properties that can help to reduce discomfort. To use herbal teas for a bruise, brew a cup of tea using the desired herb and drink it several times a day.

Herbs and techniques for reducing inflammation

Dit Da practitioners have long recognized the importance of reducing inflammation in treating injuries. Inflammation is a natural response to injury, but it can also cause pain, swelling, and stiffness that impede healing. Therefore, it is essential to address inflammation as part of a comprehensive Dit Da treatment plan. One effective way to reduce inflammation is through the use of herbal remedies and techniques.

Herbs have been used for centuries in traditional Chinese medicine to treat inflammation. One of the most common herbs used for this purpose is licorice root. Licorice root contains glycyrrhizin, which has been shown to have anti-inflammatory properties. Licorice root can be taken orally in the form of a tea or as an ingredient in herbal plasters or liniments. Another herb commonly used for reducing inflammation is turmeric. Turmeric contains curcumin, which has also been shown to have anti-inflammatory properties. Turmeric can be consumed in food or taken as a supplement.

In addition to herbal remedies, there are also techniques that can help reduce inflammation. One such technique is cupping. Cupping involves creating suction on the skin to increase blood flow and promote healing. Cupping can be used on its own or in combination with other Dit Da techniques. Another technique for reducing inflammation is acupressure. Acupressure involves applying pressure to specific points on the body to stimulate healing. Acupressure can be performed by a trained practitioner or by using self-massage techniques.

Another important aspect of reducing inflammation is rest and recovery. Resting the injured area is essential for allowing the body to heal. This may involve taking time off from physical activity or modifying activities to avoid exacerbating the injury. Rest should be balanced with gentle movement and exercise, which can help promote circulation and prevent stiffness.

Diet is another crucial factor in reducing inflammation. Certain foods have been shown to have anti-inflammatory properties, including fruits, vegetables, whole grains, and fatty fish. On the other hand, processed foods, sugar, and excessive alcohol consumption can exacerbate inflammation.

Chapter Thirteen

Sprains and Strains

Sprains and strains are common injuries that can occur as a result of physical activity or trauma. A sprain is an injury to a ligament, while a strain is an injury to a muscle or tendon. Both types of injuries can be painful and can significantly impact a person's mobility and quality of life. Fortunately, there are a variety of strategies that can be employed in Dit Da therapy to treat these injuries effectively.

One of the primary goals in treating sprains and strains is to reduce pain and inflammation. Ice can be applied to the injured area to reduce swelling and pain. Rest and elevation of the affected limb can also help to reduce inflammation. However, it is essential to balance rest with gentle movement to prevent stiffness and promote circulation. Dit Da practitioners may also recommend herbal remedies or topical treatments to reduce inflammation and promote healing. For example, herbal plasters or liniments may be applied to the affected area to reduce pain and inflammation.

Another essential aspect of treating sprains and strains is addressing any imbalances in the affected area. Injuries can disrupt the body's natural alignment, which can lead to compensatory movements and further injury. In some cases, bone-setting techniques may be employed to realign bones and joints that have been displaced by the injury. Acupressure or massage techniques may also be used to release tension in affected muscles and promote healing.

It is also crucial to address any underlying factors that may have contributed to the injury. For example, overuse injuries may be caused by poor technique or an imbalance in muscle strength. In these cases, a Dit Da practitioner may recommend corrective exercises or modifications to an individual's training routine. Additionally, a healthy diet and adequate hydration can help to support healing and prevent future injuries.

Recovery from sprains and strains can vary depending on the severity of the injury. In some cases, complete rest may be necessary, while in other cases, modified activity may be possible. Gradual return to activity is essential to prevent reinjury and promote full recovery. Physical therapy or other rehabilitation strategies may be recommended to help individuals regain strength and mobility in the affected area.

The difference between sprains and strains

Sprains and strains are two common types of injuries that can occur in the body. While these injuries share some similarities, they also have distinct differences. In Dit Da therapy, it is essential to understand the differences between sprains and strains to develop an effective treatment plan.

A sprain is an injury to a ligament, which is a tough, fibrous band of tissue that connects bone to bone. Ligaments provide stability to joints and help to prevent excessive movement. Sprains can occur when a ligament is stretched or torn beyond its normal range of motion. This can happen as a result of a sudden impact, twisting or turning, or overuse. Common sites of sprains include the ankle, knee, and wrist.

Symptoms of a sprain may include pain, swelling, bruising, and difficulty moving the affected joint. The severity of a sprain can range from mild to severe, depending on the extent of ligament damage. Mild sprains may only require rest, ice, compression, and elevation (RICE) to heal, while more severe sprains may require immobilization with a cast or brace and physical therapy to regain strength and mobility.

A strain, on the other hand, is an injury to a muscle or tendon, which is the fibrous tissue that connects muscle to bone. Strains can occur when a muscle or tendon is stretched or torn beyond its capacity. This can happen as a result of sudden or forceful movements, overuse, or improper lifting techniques. Common sites of strains include the back, hamstring, and shoulder.

Symptoms of a strain may include pain, swelling, stiffness, and difficulty moving the affected muscle or joint. The severity of a strain can range from mild to severe, depending on the extent of muscle or tendon damage. Mild strains may only require rest and gentle stretching to heal, while more severe strains may require immobilization and physical therapy to regain strength and mobility.

In Dit Da therapy, the treatment for sprains and strains may be similar in some respects, such as rest, ice, and herbal remedies to reduce pain and inflammation. However, the specific treatment strategies may differ depending on the location and severity of the injury. For example, bone-setting techniques may be used to address a sprain that has caused a bone to become displaced. Massage or acupressure techniques may be used to release tension in a strained muscle and promote healing.

In some cases, a combination of sprain and strain may occur. This can happen when a ligament and muscle or tendon are injured simultaneously. In these cases, a comprehensive treatment plan that addresses both types of injuries may be necessary.

The stages of healing and appropriate

Dit

Da treatments

Dit Da, the Chinese art of bone-setting, massage, and herbal remedies, has been used for centuries to treat a wide range of injuries, including sprains and strains. Proper treatment of these types of injuries is important to ensure proper healing and to prevent long-term damage to the affected area. Below we will discuss the stages of healing and appropriate Dit Da treatments for sprains and strains.

The first stage of healing for sprains and strains is the acute stage, which lasts for the first few days after the injury. During this stage, the focus is on reducing pain, inflammation, and swelling. To do this, Dit Da practitioners often use topical herbal remedies such as liniments, plasters, and poultices, which contain herbs such as frankincense, myrrh, and dragon's blood. These herbs are known for their ability to reduce inflammation and promote blood flow, which can help to speed up the healing process.

Another technique used during this stage is ice therapy, which involves applying ice to the affected area for 10-15 minutes at a time, several times a day. Ice therapy helps to reduce pain and swelling, and can also help to prevent further damage to the affected area.

The second stage of healing for sprains and strains is the sub-acute stage, which lasts for several days to several weeks after the injury. During this stage, the focus is on restoring range of motion and flexibility to the affected area. This is achieved through a combination of massage, stretching, and exercise.

Dit Da practitioners often use Tui Na massage techniques during this stage, which involve deep tissue massage, acupressure, and joint mobilization. These techniques can help to release tension and adhesions in the affected area, which can help to restore range of motion and flexibility.

Stretching exercises are also an important part of the sub-acute stage of healing. These exercises help to improve flexibility and mobility in the affected area, which can help to prevent further injury and promote healing.

The final stage of healing for sprains and strains is the chronic stage, which can last for several weeks to several months after the injury. During this stage, the focus is on strengthening the affected area and preventing future injuries.

Dit Da practitioners often use herbal remedies during this stage, which contain herbs such as astragalus, ginseng, and rehmannia. These herbs are known for their ability to promote healing and strengthen the body's immune system.

In addition to herbal remedies, exercises that focus on strengthening the affected area are also important during the chronic stage of healing. These exercises may include resistance training, balance training, and functional movements that mimic everyday activities.

Chapter Fourteen

Fractures and Dislocations

Fractures and dislocations are common injuries that occur in many different activities, including sports, martial arts, and everyday life. These injuries can be debilitating and require proper medical attention to heal properly. In Chinese medicine, Dit Da is the traditional practice of treating injuries, including fractures and dislocations, through a combination of herbal medicine, massage, and other therapeutic techniques.

Fractures occur when a bone is broken or cracked, and dislocations occur when a joint is forced out of its normal position. Both injuries can cause severe pain, swelling, and immobility. In traditional Chinese medicine, fractures and dislocations are seen as a disruption of the flow of Qi, or energy, in the affected area. The goal of Dit Da therapy is to restore the flow of Qi and promote the body's natural healing process.

In the case of fractures, it is important to immobilize the affected area to prevent further damage and promote proper healing. In Chinese medicine, herbs and other remedies are used to speed up the healing process and promote bone growth. Dit Da practitioners often use a combination of herbal plasters, liniments, and other topical remedies to help reduce inflammation, relieve pain, and promote healing. Common ingredients used in these remedies include frankincense, myrrh, and turmeric, which are known for their anti-inflammatory and pain-relieving properties.

In addition to topical remedies, Dit Da practitioners also use massage and acupuncture to promote the flow of Qi and stimulate the body's natural healing response. Tui Na massage is often used to help relieve muscle tension and promote circulation in the affected area. Acupuncture is also commonly used to help restore the flow of Qi and promote healing.

Dislocations require immediate attention to prevent further damage to the joint and surrounding tissues. In traditional Chinese medicine, dislocations are seen as a blockage of Qi in the affected joint. Dit Da practitioners use a combination of massage and acupuncture to restore the flow of Qi and help the joint return to its proper position. Cupping therapy is also commonly used to help relieve pain and reduce inflammation in the affected area.

After a fracture or dislocation, it is important to give the affected area time to heal properly. This may involve immobilization through the use of a cast or brace, and physical therapy to help rebuild strength and mobility. In addition, Dit Da practitioners may recommend specific exercises or stretches to help promote healing and prevent future injuries.

It is important to note that while Dit Da therapy can be effective in treating fractures and dislocations, it is not a substitute for proper medical care. In severe cases, surgery may be necessary to properly repair the affected area. However, Dit Da therapy can be used in conjunction with medical treatment to help promote healing and reduce pain and inflammation.

Assessing and managing fractures and dislocations

Fractures and dislocations are common injuries that can be very painful and disabling. A fracture is a break in a bone, while a dislocation is a displacement of a bone from its normal position. These injuries can occur from a variety of causes, such as falls, sports injuries, and car accidents.

When someone sustains a fracture or dislocation, it is important to properly assess and manage the injury to ensure the best possible outcome. In Dit Da therapy, this involves a combination of physical examination, imaging tests, and treatment techniques that are specific to each individual case.

The first step in assessing a fracture or dislocation is a thorough physical examination. The injured area will be inspected for signs of deformity, swelling, and discoloration. The range of motion and strength of the affected limb or joint will also be evaluated. The practitioner will ask the patient to describe their pain and other symptoms, such as numbness or tingling. In some cases, imaging tests such as X-rays or CT scans may be ordered to confirm the diagnosis and assess the severity of the injury.

Once the injury has been properly diagnosed, the next step is to manage the pain and swelling. This may involve applying ice packs, compression bandages, and elevating the injured limb. Pain medication may also be prescribed as needed.

In Dit Da therapy, there are several techniques that can be used to accelerate the healing process and promote proper bone and joint alignment. One of the most common techniques is bone setting, which involves manipulating the broken bone back into its proper position. This is often done using gentle pressure and manipulation, with the goal of reducing pain and swelling and promoting proper healing.

Another technique that can be used in Dit Da therapy is moxibustion, which involves burning dried herbs close to the skin to stimulate healing and reduce pain. This technique can be especially effective for treating bone fractures, as it can help to increase blood flow to the affected area and promote bone growth.

Herbal plasters and liniments can also be used in Dit Da therapy to reduce swelling and inflammation, and promote healing. These may include a variety of herbs and other natural ingredients, such as camphor, menthol, and eucalyptus oil. These plasters and liniments are often applied directly to the injured area, and may be covered with a bandage or wrap to help them stay in place.

In addition to these techniques, it is also important to maintain proper nutrition and hydration during the healing process. This can help to provide the body with the nutrients it needs to promote healing and recovery, and can also help to prevent further injury.

Recovery and rehabilitation techniques

Recovery and rehabilitation are essential for patients who have suffered from injuries. The road to recovery can be long and arduous, but with the proper techniques, it can be made easier. This is where Dit Da therapy comes in. Dit Da, a traditional Chinese medicine practice, has been used for centuries to treat injuries and promote healing.

The first step in recovery and rehabilitation is rest. Injuries need time to heal, and overexertion can cause further damage. Proper rest allows the body to focus its energy on healing the injury. Dit Da therapy emphasizes the importance of rest and relaxation in the recovery process.

Once the initial pain and swelling have subsided, it is important to begin gentle movement and exercises. This promotes circulation, which helps to bring healing nutrients and oxygen to the injured area. Dit Da practitioners often use Qi Gong and Tui Na massage to gently stimulate circulation in the injured area.

In addition to movement, proper nutrition is also important for recovery. The body needs a variety of nutrients to heal and rebuild injured tissues. Dit Da practitioners often prescribe herbal remedies and dietary changes to support the healing process. For example, foods high in vitamin C can promote collagen production, which is essential for the formation of new tissues.

As the injured area continues to heal, it is important to gradually increase the intensity of exercises and activities. This helps to rebuild strength and flexibility in the injured area. However, it is important to do this gradually and under the guidance of a qualified practitioner to avoid reinjury.

In some cases, a patient may benefit from more specialized treatments such as acupuncture or cupping therapy. Acupuncture can help to reduce pain and inflammation, while cupping therapy can help to promote circulation and release tension in the muscles and connective tissues.

It is important to note that recovery and rehabilitation are not always straightforward. Each injury and each patient is unique, and the road to recovery can vary greatly depending on many factors. A qualified Dit Da practitioner will work with each patient to create a customized treatment plan that takes into account their individual needs and circumstances.

In addition to physical healing, it is also important to address the emotional and psychological aspects of recovery. Injuries can be stressful and traumatic, and patients may experience anxiety or depression as a result. Dit Da therapy takes a holistic approach to healing, addressing both the physical and emotional aspects of recovery.

Chapter Fifteen

Internal Injuries

Dit Da is a traditional Chinese medicine practice that has been used for centuries to treat various types of injuries, including internal injuries. Internal injuries, also known as "nei jin" in Chinese, refer to damage to internal organs or tissues caused by physical trauma or other factors. These injuries can be serious and may require immediate medical attention, but Dit Da can also be used to help alleviate symptoms and promote healing.

1. The key to treating internal injuries with Dit Da is to identify the specific type of injury and its underlying causes. This requires a thorough understanding of the anatomy and physiology of the affected area, as well as the principles of Chinese medicine. In general, internal injuries can be classified into three main categories: Qi deficiency, Qi stagnation, and blood stasis.

Qi deficiency refers to a lack of energy or vitality in the affected area, which can lead to weakness, fatigue, and poor circulation. This type of injury is often caused by chronic stress or overwork, and may be treated with tonifying herbs and acupuncture points that help to replenish Qi and promote circulation.

Qi stagnation, on the other hand, refers to a blockage or obstruction of Qi flow in the affected area, which can cause pain, inflammation, and swelling. This type of injury is often caused by acute trauma or emotional stress, and may be treated with herbs and acupuncture points that help to move Qi and promote circulation.

Blood stasis refers to a blockage or stagnation of blood flow in the affected area, which can lead to pain, inflammation, and tissue damage. This type of injury is often caused by physical trauma or chronic inflammation, and may be treated with herbs and acupuncture points that help to promote blood circulation and remove blood stasis.

In addition to herbal remedies and acupuncture, Dit Da may also involve the use of massage, cupping, and moxibustion to help alleviate symptoms and promote healing. Massage can be used to stimulate circulation and promote lymphatic drainage in the affected area, while cupping and moxibustion can be used to promote blood flow and reduce inflammation.

It is important to note that while Dit Da can be effective in treating internal injuries, it should not be used as a substitute for proper medical care. If you suspect that you have suffered an internal injury, it is important to seek medical attention immediately to ensure proper diagnosis and treatment.

Recognizing and treating internal injuries

Dit Da medicine is a traditional Chinese system of healing that utilizes various techniques and remedies to treat injuries, both internal and external. While external injuries such as bruises, sprains, and fractures are more commonly associated with Dit Da, the system is also effective in treating internal injuries such as organ damage, internal bleeding, and nerve damage.

Internal injuries can be difficult to diagnose and treat, as they are not always visible or immediately apparent. They may result from a variety of causes, including blunt force trauma, falls, and accidents. Injuries to the internal organs can be particularly dangerous, as they may lead to serious complications or even death if left untreated.

The first step in recognizing and treating internal injuries is to understand the symptoms and signs associated with these types of injuries. Symptoms of internal injuries can vary widely depending on the nature and severity of the injury, but some common signs to look out for include pain or discomfort in the affected area, swelling, bruising, and difficulty breathing or moving. If the injury is located in the abdominal region, symptoms may include nausea, vomiting, and abdominal pain.

Once an internal injury has been identified, it is important to seek medical attention immediately. While Dit Da medicine can be effective in treating internal injuries, it is not a replacement for modern medical care. In some cases, surgery or other medical interventions may be necessary to address the injury.

In addition to seeking medical care, a number of Dit Da techniques and remedies may be used to help manage and heal internal injuries. Acupuncture and moxibustion, for example, can help to reduce inflammation and promote healing. These techniques involve the insertion of fine needles or the application of heat to specific points on the body. This can help to stimulate blood flow and promote the body's natural healing processes.

Herbal remedies may also be used to treat internal injuries. Many of the same herbs used in Dit Da medicine for external injuries may also be effective for internal injuries. For example, herbs such as arnica and comfrey may be used to reduce inflammation and promote healing. In addition, certain herbs such as ginseng and astragalus may help to strengthen the body and promote overall health.

Diet and lifestyle changes may also play an important role in treating internal injuries. Eating a healthy diet rich in fruits, vegetables, and whole grains can help to support the body's natural healing processes. Additionally, getting plenty of rest and avoiding activities that may aggravate the injury can help to speed up the healing process.

It is important to note that the treatment of internal injuries with Dit Da medicine should always be done under the guidance of a qualified practitioner. While many of the techniques and remedies used in Dit Da medicine are safe and effective, they can also be harmful if used incorrectly or without proper training.

The role of

Dit

Da in healing internal damage

The ancient Chinese healing art of Dit Da, also known as "hit medicine," has been used for centuries to treat a wide range of injuries, including internal damage. Dit Da practitioners understand the importance of addressing internal injuries, as these can often be more serious and debilitating than external injuries.

Internal injuries can result from a variety of causes, including trauma from blunt force, such as from a fall or car accident, or from more subtle forces, such as stress or emotional trauma. Common internal injuries include bruising, organ damage, and muscle or tissue tears. These injuries can lead to pain, inflammation, and reduced organ function.

The first step in treating internal injuries with Dit Da is to accurately diagnose the injury. This requires a thorough examination by a trained practitioner who is skilled in palpation and observation. The practitioner will assess the affected area, looking for signs of swelling, tenderness, and discoloration. They will also ask about the patient's medical history and any previous injuries.

Once a diagnosis is made, the practitioner will develop a treatment plan tailored to the specific injury. This may include the use of herbal remedies, acupuncture, cupping, and moxibustion. The practitioner may also recommend dietary and lifestyle changes to support the healing process.

Herbal remedies are a cornerstone of Dit Da therapy for internal injuries. Many herbs have been found to have anti-inflammatory and pain-relieving properties, making them effective in treating internal damage. Some commonly used herbs include arnica, turmeric, ginger, and frankincense.

Acupuncture is another important tool in the Dit Da practitioner's arsenal for treating internal injuries. Acupuncture works by stimulating specific points along the body's meridian system, which helps to balance the body's energy and promote healing. This can be particularly helpful in cases of organ damage, as it can improve organ function and reduce inflammation.

Cupping is another technique that can be effective in treating internal injuries. Cupping involves placing cups on the skin and creating suction, which can help to promote blood flow and reduce inflammation. This technique can be particularly effective for bruising and tissue damage.

Moxibustion, which involves burning dried herbs on specific points on the body, can also be helpful in treating internal injuries. Moxibustion is thought to improve circulation and reduce inflammation, making it effective in treating a wide range of injuries.

In addition to these techniques, Dit Da practitioners may also recommend dietary and lifestyle changes to support healing. This may include avoiding certain foods, such as alcohol and processed foods, and incorporating more nutrient-dense foods, such as leafy greens and lean protein. The practitioner may also recommend stress-reduction techniques, such as meditation or tai chi, to support the healing process.

Chapter Sixteen

Chronic Pain Management

Chronic pain is a common health condition affecting millions of people around the world. It is characterized by persistent pain that lasts for more than 3 months, and it can be caused by a variety of factors such as injury, disease, and nerve damage. Chronic pain can significantly affect an individual's quality of life, causing physical and emotional distress, and limiting their daily activities. While there are various medical treatments available for chronic pain management, traditional Chinese medicine offers a holistic approach that can be effective in managing chronic pain. One of the most effective methods in traditional Chinese medicine for managing chronic pain is Dit Da therapy.

Dit Da therapy is a traditional Chinese medicine technique used for healing bruises, sprains, fractures, and other injuries. It is a combination of herbal remedies, acupuncture, cupping, and massage. The technique focuses on restoring the balance of energy and blood flow in the body, which helps to reduce inflammation and promote healing.

Dit Da therapy can be used for chronic pain management as well. Chronic pain is often caused by blockages in the body's energy channels, which leads to reduced blood flow and the accumulation of toxins in the affected area. By restoring the balance of energy and blood flow, Dit Da therapy can help to reduce inflammation and relieve pain.

One of the key components of Dit Da therapy for chronic pain management is acupuncture. Acupuncture is a traditional Chinese medicine technique that involves the insertion of fine needles into specific points on the body. These points correspond to energy channels in the body, and the insertion of needles helps to stimulate the flow of energy and blood, which helps to relieve pain and promote healing. Acupuncture is an effective treatment for chronic pain, and it is often used in conjunction with other traditional Chinese medicine techniques such as herbal remedies and massage.

Another important component of Dit Da therapy for chronic pain management is herbal remedies. Chinese herbs have been used for centuries to treat a wide range of health conditions, including chronic pain. The herbs used in Dit Da therapy are carefully selected based on their properties and the specific needs of the patient. Herbal remedies can be taken orally or applied topically, and they work by reducing inflammation, promoting circulation, and relieving pain.

Cupping is another technique used in Dit Da therapy for chronic pain management. Cupping involves the use of special cups that are placed on the skin and suctioned to create a vacuum. This vacuum helps to stimulate blood flow and promote healing. Cupping is particularly effective for treating chronic pain in the back and neck, and it is often used in conjunction with massage and acupuncture.

Massage is also an important component of Dit Da therapy for chronic pain management. Massage helps to relieve tension in the muscles and promote circulation, which helps to reduce inflammation and relieve pain. There are various massage techniques used in Dit Da therapy, including Tui Na massage, which involves the use of pressure and stretching to promote healing.

In addition to these techniques, there are various lifestyle changes that can help to manage chronic pain. These include maintaining a healthy diet, getting regular exercise, and practicing stress-reduction techniques such as meditation and yoga. By adopting a holistic approach to chronic pain management that includes traditional Chinese medicine techniques such as Dit Da therapy, individuals can effectively manage their pain and improve their overall quality of life.

Addressing chronic pain with

Dit

Da therapy

Dit Da therapy, which is a traditional Chinese medicine technique, has been used for centuries to treat various kinds of pain. It is a holistic approach that involves the use of different modalities, including herbal remedies, massage, acupuncture, and others, to address pain at its root cause. Below we will explore how Dit Da therapy can be used to address chronic pain.

Chronic pain is defined as pain that lasts for longer than three months. It can have many causes, including injuries, arthritis, fibromyalgia, and nerve damage. Chronic pain can be debilitating, affecting a person's quality of life, ability to work, and overall health. Many people turn to pain medication to manage chronic pain, but this approach can be problematic, as it can lead to addiction, tolerance, and other side effects.

Dit Da therapy offers an alternative approach to managing chronic pain. Rather than masking the symptoms of pain, it aims to address the underlying causes of pain. This can involve identifying and treating imbalances in the body, promoting circulation, reducing inflammation, and supporting the body's natural healing processes.

One of the key components of Dit Da therapy for chronic pain is the use of herbal remedies. Herbal remedies have been used for thousands of years to treat a wide range of health conditions, including pain. There are many different herbs that can be used for pain, including ginger, turmeric, willow bark, and others. These herbs have natural anti-inflammatory properties, which can help to reduce pain and inflammation in the body.

Another important component of Dit Da therapy for chronic pain is massage. Massage can be used to promote circulation, reduce tension in muscles, and release trigger points that can contribute to pain. Tui Na massage is a specific type of massage that is often used in Dit Da therapy. It involves deep tissue massage and stretching, and can be used to address a wide range of pain conditions.

Acupuncture is another modality that can be used in Dit Da therapy for chronic pain. Acupuncture involves the insertion of thin needles into specific points on the body. These points are believed to correspond to different organs and systems in the body, and by stimulating these points, acupuncture can help to balance the body and promote healing. Acupuncture has been shown to be effective for many types of pain, including back pain, neck pain, and headaches.

In addition to these modalities, there are other techniques that can be used in Dit Da therapy for chronic pain. These may include cupping, moxibustion, and gua sha. Cupping involves the use of suction cups to promote circulation and reduce pain. Moxibustion involves the use of burning herbs to warm and stimulate specific points on the body. Gua sha involves the use of a smooth-edged tool to scrape the skin and promote circulation.

Complementary therapies for pain relief

Complementary therapies are a vital aspect of pain relief and management, especially for those who have chronic pain. While Western medicine primarily focuses on pharmaceutical interventions, complementary therapies offer alternative methods of addressing pain that can be used in conjunction with or instead of medications. Among these complementary therapies is Dit Da, a traditional Chinese medicine practice that has been used for centuries to alleviate pain and promote healing. Below we will explore the role of complementary therapies, including Dit Da, in pain relief and management.

Complementary therapies aim to provide relief to individuals who experience chronic pain that may not respond well to pharmaceutical interventions. Chronic pain can be debilitating, affecting one's ability to carry out daily tasks and leading to a poor quality of life. Complementary therapies can help alleviate pain and improve a person's overall well-being, without the side effects that can be associated with medications.

Dit Da is a traditional Chinese medicine practice that uses a variety of techniques, such as acupuncture, cupping, and herbal remedies, to promote healing and alleviate pain. The practice originated in China and was traditionally used by martial artists to treat injuries sustained during training. However, it has now become a popular practice for those who experience chronic pain, as well as athletes and others who have sustained injuries.

One of the primary techniques used in Dit Da is acupuncture. Acupuncture involves inserting thin needles into specific points on the body to stimulate the flow of energy or qi. It is believed that the flow of energy can become blocked or disrupted, leading to pain and other symptoms. By stimulating specific points, acupuncture can help restore the flow of energy, promoting healing and alleviating pain.

Cupping is another technique used in Dit Da, which involves placing cups on the skin and creating a vacuum to draw the skin and underlying tissue up into the cup. This technique is believed to increase blood flow, promoting healing and reducing pain. Herbal remedies, such as topical ointments and internal herbal preparations, are also commonly used in Dit Da to promote healing and alleviate pain.

While Dit Da is a traditional Chinese medicine practice, it has gained popularity in the Western world in recent years. Many practitioners of complementary therapies offer Dit Da as a treatment option for those who experience chronic pain or injuries. In fact, many athletes, including Olympic athletes, have turned to Dit Da to help them recover from injuries sustained during training and competition.

In addition to Dit Da, there are several other complementary therapies that can be used in conjunction with or instead of medications to alleviate pain. These include massage therapy, chiropractic care, and aromatherapy, among others. Each of these therapies has its own unique benefits and can be tailored to meet the individual needs of each patient.

Massage therapy involves manipulating the soft tissues of the body to promote relaxation and alleviate pain. Chiropractic care involves manipulating the spine and joints to improve mobility and reduce pain. Aromatherapy involves using essential oils to promote relaxation and alleviate pain. These complementary therapies can be used alone or in combination with other therapies, such as medications, to provide the best possible outcomes for patients.

Chapter Seventeen

Treating Common Sports Injuries

Sports injuries are a common occurrence among athletes, ranging from minor strains to severe fractures. Injuries can happen during training, competition, or even casual activities. Many athletes turn to Dit Da therapy to aid in the healing process and manage their pain. Dit Da therapy, which is also known as "hit medicine," originated in ancient China and is a combination of massage, herbal remedies, and acupuncture. Below we will explore the techniques and methods of Dit Da therapy in treating common sports injuries.

One of the most common sports injuries is a strain, which occurs when a muscle or tendon is overstretched or torn. This type of injury can cause swelling, pain, and limited mobility. Dit Da therapy can help reduce inflammation and improve circulation in the affected area. Herbal plasters and liniments can be applied topically to the injured area to provide relief from pain and reduce inflammation. Acupuncture can also be used to target specific areas and stimulate the body's natural healing process.

Another common sports injury is a sprain, which occurs when ligaments are stretched or torn. This type of injury can be particularly painful and can lead to long-term damage if left untreated. Similar to strains, Dit Da therapy can help reduce inflammation and improve circulation to the affected area. Cupping therapy can be particularly effective in treating sprains. This technique involves placing a heated cup over the injured area, creating suction, which can help improve circulation and reduce pain.

Fractures and dislocations are also common sports injuries, particularly among athletes who engage in high-impact sports. These types of injuries require immediate medical attention, but Dit Da therapy can also aid in the recovery process. Acupuncture can help reduce pain and inflammation and promote the body's natural healing process. Herbal remedies, such as moxibustion, can also be used to improve blood flow to the injured area and speed up the healing process.

In addition to treating specific injuries, Dit Da therapy can also help athletes manage chronic pain. Chronic pain is a common issue among athletes, particularly those who engage in repetitive movements, such as runners or swimmers. Cupping therapy and acupuncture can be particularly effective in managing chronic pain. These techniques can help improve circulation and promote the release of endorphins, which are natural painkillers.

It's important to note that while Dit Da therapy can be effective in treating sports injuries, it should not be used as a substitute for medical treatment. If you experience a severe injury, it's important to seek medical attention immediately. Dit Da therapy can be used in conjunction with medical treatment to aid in the healing process and manage pain.

Applying

Dit

Da principles to sports injuries

Dit Da therapy, also known as the "hit medicine," is a traditional Chinese medicine technique that has been used for centuries to treat injuries caused by martial arts, sports, and other physical activities. It involves a combination of manual techniques, herbal remedies, and dietary changes to promote healing and reduce pain. Below we will explore how Dit Da principles can be applied to common sports injuries.

One of the most common sports injuries is a sprain, which occurs when a ligament is stretched or torn. The first step in treating a sprain is to rest the affected area and apply ice to reduce inflammation. In Dit Da therapy, topical herbal remedies such as Zheng Gu Shui or Tieh Ta Yao Gin can be applied to the affected area to reduce pain and promote healing. These remedies typically contain ingredients such as camphor, menthol, and arnica, which have anti-inflammatory and pain-relieving properties.

Another common sports injury is a strain, which occurs when a muscle or tendon is stretched or torn. Rest and ice are also important for treating strains, but massage therapy can also be beneficial. Tui Na massage is a form of Chinese massage that can be used to promote circulation and reduce muscle tension, helping to speed up the healing process. Cupping therapy, another technique used in Dit Da therapy, can also be used to reduce pain and inflammation associated with strains.

Fractures are less common but can be more severe sports injuries. In these cases, immediate medical attention is necessary. However, after the initial treatment, Dit Da therapy can be used to promote healing and reduce pain. Acupuncture can be used to stimulate circulation and reduce inflammation, while moxibustion can be used to promote the healing of bone fractures. Herbal remedies, such as Gui Zhi Fu Ling Wan or Shu Jing Huo Xue Wan, can also be used to promote bone healing and reduce pain.

In addition to the specific techniques used in Dit Da therapy, there are also general principles that can be applied to sports injuries. One important principle is the use of both heat and cold therapy. Cold therapy is typically used immediately after an injury to reduce inflammation and pain, while heat therapy can be used later on to promote circulation and relaxation of the affected area. In Dit Da therapy, moxibustion and herbal plasters can be used for heat therapy, while ice or cold water can be used for cold therapy.

Another important principle is the use of rest and proper nutrition. Rest is important for allowing the body to heal, and proper nutrition is important for providing the body with the nutrients it needs to support the healing process. In Dit Da therapy, dietary changes may be recommended to promote healing, such as consuming foods that are high in protein and vitamin C, which are important for tissue repair and immune function.

Prevention and recovery strategies

Injuries are an unfortunate but common occurrence in the world of sports. From minor sprains and strains to more serious fractures and dislocations, athletes are susceptible to a wide range of injuries that can significantly impact their performance and even end their careers. However, with the right prevention and recovery strategies, many of these injuries can be avoided or at least minimized. One such strategy is the use of Dit Da therapy, an ancient Chinese form of healing that has been used for centuries to treat injuries and promote overall health and wellness.

Dit Da, which literally means "hit and fall," is a branch of traditional Chinese medicine that focuses specifically on the treatment of trauma injuries. It encompasses a wide range of techniques and modalities, including acupuncture, cupping, moxibustion, gua sha, herbal remedies, and massage. The goal of Dit Da therapy is to promote the flow of qi (energy) and blood throughout the body, which in turn helps to facilitate the healing process.

One of the key principles of Dit Da therapy is prevention. By taking steps to prevent injuries from occurring in the first place, athletes can significantly reduce their risk of developing chronic pain or suffering from more serious injuries. Some of the most effective prevention strategies include proper warm-up and cool-down techniques, stretching and flexibility exercises, strength training, and wearing appropriate protective gear.

However, despite their best efforts, athletes may still experience injuries from time to time. In these cases, Dit Da therapy can be a valuable tool in helping to facilitate the healing process and speed up recovery time. One of the most common Dit Da techniques used for sports injuries is massage. By applying pressure to the affected area, massage can help to increase blood flow and promote the release of endorphins, which can help to reduce pain and improve mood.

Another common Dit Da technique is cupping, which involves using cups to create suction on the skin. Cupping can be particularly effective in treating muscle strains and sprains, as it helps to improve circulation and reduce inflammation. Moxibustion, which involves burning an herb called mugwort close to the skin, is also commonly used in Dit Da therapy to help reduce pain and promote healing.

Herbal remedies are another important component of Dit Da therapy. Depending on the specific injury, different herbs may be used to help promote healing and reduce pain and inflammation. Some of the most commonly used herbs in Dit Da therapy include arnica, comfrey, and yarrow.

In addition to these techniques and modalities, athletes can also benefit from incorporating other complementary therapies into their recovery plan. For example, acupuncture, which involves the insertion of thin needles into specific points on the body, has been shown to be effective in reducing pain and promoting healing. Yoga and tai chi, two practices that focus on breath control and gentle movement, can also be helpful in reducing stress and improving overall physical and mental well-being.

While Dit Da therapy can be effective in treating a wide range of sports injuries, it is important to remember that it is just one component of a comprehensive recovery plan. Depending on the severity of the injury, athletes may also need to undergo more traditional medical treatments, such as surgery or physical therapy. However, by incorporating Dit Da therapy into their overall recovery plan, athletes can help to promote faster healing, reduce pain and inflammation, and get back to their sport more quickly.

Chapter Eighteen

Integrating Dit Da into Daily Life

Integrating Dit Da into daily life can be a great way to maintain and improve overall health and wellbeing. Dit Da is a traditional Chinese therapeutic practice that has been used for centuries to treat various types of injuries, such as bruises, sprains, and strains. However, its benefits go beyond just treating injuries. By incorporating Dit Da principles into daily life, individuals can improve their physical and mental health, increase their energy levels, and reduce stress and tension.

One way to integrate Dit Da into daily life is by practicing Qi Gong. Qi Gong is a series of gentle exercises that combine breathing techniques with slow, flowing movements. This practice is designed to improve the flow of Qi, or life force energy, throughout the body. By practicing Qi Gong regularly, individuals can improve their overall health, increase their energy levels, and reduce stress and tension. Qi Gong exercises can be done at any time of day and can be easily incorporated into a daily routine.

Another way to integrate Dit Da into daily life is by using acupressure techniques. Acupressure is a technique that involves applying pressure to specific points on the body to stimulate the flow of Qi. By using acupressure regularly, individuals can improve their overall health and wellbeing. Acupressure can be easily incorporated into a daily routine, such as applying pressure to specific acupressure points while sitting at a desk or during a break from work.

Herbal remedies can also be integrated into daily life to promote health and wellbeing. There are many different herbs that can be used in Dit Da therapy to treat various ailments, such as ginger, turmeric, and ginseng. By incorporating these herbs into daily meals or consuming them in the form of tea or supplements, individuals can improve their overall health and reduce the risk of illness.

Meditation is another way to integrate Dit Da into daily life. Meditation involves focusing the mind and achieving a state of calm and relaxation. By practicing meditation regularly, individuals can reduce stress and tension, improve their mental clarity, and increase their overall sense of wellbeing. Meditation can be easily incorporated into a daily routine, such as taking a few minutes to meditate before or after work or before going to bed.

Stretching and mobility exercises can also be incorporated into daily life to promote overall health and wellbeing. By stretching and mobilizing the body regularly, individuals can improve their flexibility and range of motion, reduce the risk of injury, and improve their overall physical health.

In addition to these practices, individuals can also incorporate Dit Da into their daily life by adopting a healthy diet, getting regular exercise, and getting adequate sleep. Eating a healthy diet that is rich in nutrients can provide the body with the fuel it needs to function properly. Regular exercise can help to maintain and improve physical health, while adequate sleep can help to reduce stress and tension and improve mental clarity.

Creating a

Dit

Da self-care routine

Dit Da, or "hit medicine," is a traditional Chinese healing art that has been used for centuries to treat martial arts injuries and other forms of trauma. Its techniques include herbal remedies, massage, acupuncture, and other modalities, all of which can be applied to create a comprehensive self-care routine that promotes wellness, prevents injury, and speeds recovery from both physical and emotional stress.

Creating a Dit Da self-care routine begins with developing an awareness of one's body and its needs. This means paying attention to warning signs of injury, such as pain, stiffness, or limited mobility, and taking steps to address them before they become more serious. It also involves adopting healthy habits, such as good posture, regular exercise, and a balanced diet, that support the body's natural healing processes.

One of the key principles of Dit Da is the importance of stimulating the body's natural energy, or Qi, to promote healing and balance. This can be done through a variety of exercises, such as Qigong, Tai Chi, or Yoga, that focus on deep breathing, gentle movement, and relaxation. These practices help to increase circulation, reduce stress, and enhance the body's natural ability to heal itself.

Another important aspect of a Dit Da self-care routine is the use of herbal remedies, such as liniments, poultices, and teas, to soothe pain, reduce inflammation, and promote healing. These remedies are typically made from a combination of natural herbs, such as ginseng, ginger, and arnica, that have been used for centuries to treat a wide range of ailments. They can be applied topically, taken orally, or used in combination with other therapies, such as acupuncture or massage.

Massage is another important component of a Dit Da self-care routine, as it helps to increase circulation, relieve tension, and reduce pain. Techniques such as Tui Na, Gua Sha, and Cupping are often used to stimulate the body's natural healing processes, loosen tight muscles, and promote relaxation. These techniques can be done by a trained practitioner or self-administered using a variety of tools, such as massage balls, rollers, and foam rollers.

Acupuncture is another powerful tool for promoting health and wellness, as it helps to balance the body's energy and stimulate its natural healing processes. This ancient Chinese therapy involves the insertion of fine needles into specific points on the body, which helps to stimulate the release of endorphins and other natural pain-relieving chemicals. It can be used to treat a wide range of conditions, from chronic pain to anxiety and depression.

In addition to these techniques, there are a number of other practices that can be incorporated into a Dit Da self-care routine, such as meditation, visualization, and affirmations. These practices help to reduce stress, increase focus, and promote a positive mindset, which can have a profound impact on overall health and wellness.

Tips for maintaining a healthy lifestyle

Maintaining a healthy lifestyle is essential for overall well-being, and it can also help prevent certain health conditions. The practice of Dit Da therapy, which involves the use of natural remedies and techniques for treating injuries and promoting healing, can be a valuable addition to a healthy lifestyle. Here are some tips for incorporating Dit Da principles into your daily routine:

1. Practice good nutrition: Proper nutrition is essential for maintaining good health, and it can also help support the body's natural healing process. Include plenty of fresh fruits and vegetables, lean protein sources,

and whole grains in your diet. Avoid processed foods, excess sugar, and unhealthy fats.

2. Exercise regularly: Exercise is crucial for maintaining physical fitness and can also help reduce the risk of certain health conditions. Incorporate regular exercise into your routine, including strength training, cardio, and flexibility exercises.

3. Practice stress-reduction techniques: Stress can negatively impact physical and mental health, so it is important to find ways to manage it. Techniques like meditation, deep breathing, and yoga can help reduce stress and promote relaxation.

4. Get plenty of rest: Adequate sleep is crucial for overall health, and it is also important for promoting healing and injury recovery. Aim for 7-9 hours of sleep per night and establish a regular sleep routine.

5. Use natural remedies: Incorporate natural remedies like herbal teas, essential oils, and topical ointments into your routine for preventing and treating injuries. For example, ginger tea can help reduce inflammation and soreness, while arnica ointment can be applied topically to reduce pain and swelling.

6. Prioritize injury prevention: While injuries can happen to anyone, there are steps you can take to reduce your risk. Warm up before exercising, use proper form and technique, and wear appropriate protective gear.

7. Address injuries promptly: If you do experience an injury, seek medical attention as soon as possible. Use natural remedies like Dit Da formulas to support the body's natural healing process and promote faster recovery.

By incorporating these tips into your daily routine, you can create a healthy lifestyle that supports injury prevention and promotes overall well-being. The principles of Dit Da therapy can be a valuable addition to your self-care routine, helping to promote healing and injury recovery naturally and effectively.

Chapter Nineteen

Dit Da for Emotional Well-being

Dit Da, also known as bone-setting, is a Chinese healing technique that has been used for thousands of years to treat physical injuries and pain. However, many people are not aware of the potential benefits of Dit Da for emotional well-being. Below we will explore the connection between Dit Da and emotional health, and discuss some techniques for using Dit Da to promote overall well-being.

In traditional Chinese medicine, it is believed that physical and emotional health are closely linked. According to this philosophy, when the body is out of balance, it can lead to emotional imbalances such as anxiety, depression, and irritability. Dit Da techniques can help to restore balance to the body, which can have a positive effect on emotional well-being.

One way that Dit Da can promote emotional health is through its ability to reduce stress. Stress is a common problem in modern society, and it can have a negative impact on both physical and emotional health. By using Dit Da techniques such as acupressure and cupping, it is possible to release tension and promote relaxation in the body. This can help to reduce stress levels, which can have a positive effect on mood and overall well-being.

Another way that Dit Da can benefit emotional health is by improving the flow of Qi, or life energy, in the body. In traditional Chinese medicine, it is believed that Qi flows through the body along channels called meridians. When there is a blockage or imbalance in the flow of Qi, it can lead to physical and emotional health problems. By using Dit Da techniques such as acupuncture and moxibustion, it is possible to stimulate the flow of Qi and promote overall balance and harmony in the body.

In addition to its physical benefits, Dit Da can also have a positive effect on emotional health by promoting mindfulness and self-awareness. Many Dit Da techniques, such as Qi Gong and meditation, involve focusing the mind and becoming more aware of the present moment. By practicing these techniques regularly, it is possible to develop a greater sense of mindfulness and self-awareness, which can have a positive impact on emotional health.

If you are interested in using Dit Da to promote emotional well-being, there are several techniques that you can try. Acupressure is a simple and effective technique that involves applying pressure to specific points on the body to stimulate the flow of Qi and promote relaxation. Cupping is another technique that can be used to release tension and promote relaxation in the body. Qi Gong and meditation are also effective techniques for promoting mindfulness and self-awareness.

It is important to note that while Dit Da can be a powerful tool for promoting emotional well-being, it is not a substitute for professional mental health treatment. If you are experiencing emotional health problems, it is important to seek the help of a qualified mental health professional.

How

Dit

Da can promote emotional balance

Dit Da, a traditional Chinese medicine technique, is widely used for treating physical injuries, but it also has potential benefits for emotional well-being. Dit Da is based on the principle of Qi, which is the vital energy that flows through the body. The Qi is responsible for maintaining physical, mental, and emotional health. Any imbalance in the Qi can lead to physical and emotional ailments. By using Dit Da, one can balance the Qi to promote emotional balance.

Dit Da promotes emotional balance in various ways. Firstly, Dit Da therapy involves massage, which promotes relaxation and reduces stress. Massage increases the production of endorphins, the body's natural painkillers, and mood elevators. Endorphins are known to reduce anxiety, depression, and stress. When the body is relaxed, it reduces the production of cortisol, the stress hormone. High levels of cortisol can lead to anxiety, depression, and other emotional imbalances. Therefore, by reducing cortisol levels and increasing endorphins, Dit Da promotes emotional well-being.

Secondly, Dit Da also promotes emotional balance through the use of acupressure points. Acupressure points are specific points on the body that are believed to influence the flow of Qi. By pressing these points, one can balance the flow of Qi and promote emotional balance. For example, the acupressure point known as Pericardium 6, or Nei Guan, is located on the inner wrist and is known to promote relaxation, reduce stress, and improve sleep quality. By stimulating this point, one can promote emotional balance.

Thirdly, Dit Da incorporates the use of herbs and essential oils that have a calming effect on the body and mind. For example, lavender essential oil is known for its calming properties and can help reduce anxiety, stress, and depression. Similarly, herbs such as chamomile and valerian root have been used for centuries to promote relaxation and sleep. By incorporating these herbs and oils into Dit Da therapy, one can promote emotional balance.

Finally, Dit Da also emphasizes the importance of proper breathing techniques. Breathing exercises are known to reduce stress, promote relaxation, and improve emotional balance. By using breathing techniques such as deep breathing or belly breathing, one can calm the mind and promote emotional well-being.

Techniques for stress reduction and relaxation

Dit Da is a traditional Chinese medicine practice that involves the use of various techniques to treat injuries and promote overall health and wellness. While often associated with physical injuries, Dit Da can also be used to manage stress and promote relaxation. Below we will explore some techniques for stress reduction and relaxation within the context of Dit Da.

One of the most effective ways to reduce stress and promote relaxation is through deep breathing techniques. In Dit Da, practitioners often use a technique called "abdominal breathing," which involves breathing deeply into the abdomen rather than shallowly into the chest. This technique allows for a greater intake of oxygen and can help to calm the nervous system.

Another technique used in Dit Da for stress reduction is meditation. Meditation involves sitting quietly and focusing the mind on a specific object, thought, or activity. This practice can help to reduce stress, anxiety, and depression, and can also promote feelings of calm and relaxation. In Dit Da, practitioners may use various meditation techniques, including mindfulness meditation and visualization.

Massage therapy is another effective way to reduce stress and promote relaxation within the context of Dit Da. Massage can help to relieve muscle tension, improve circulation, and promote feelings of calm and relaxation.

In Dit Da, practitioners may use various massage techniques, including Tui Na massage, acupressure, and Gua Sha.

Herbs and essential oils can also be used in Dit Da to promote relaxation and reduce stress. Certain herbs, such as chamomile, lavender, and passionflower, have been traditionally used for their calming properties. Essential oils can be diffused or applied topically to promote relaxation and reduce stress.

Exercise is also an important component of a Dit Da practice for stress reduction and relaxation. Exercise helps to reduce stress hormones in the body and promotes the release of endorphins, which are natural mood boosters. In Dit Da, practitioners may incorporate exercises such as Qi Gong or Tai Chi, which involve slow, deliberate movements and deep breathing.

Finally, it is important to consider the role of nutrition in managing stress and promoting relaxation. A healthy diet that is rich in fruits, vegetables, whole grains, and lean protein can provide the nutrients the body needs to support overall health and wellness. In Dit Da, practitioners may recommend certain foods or supplements, such as green tea or adaptogenic herbs like ashwagandha or Rhodiola rosea, which have been shown to have stress-reducing properties.

Chapter Twenty

Becoming a Dit Da Practitioner

Dit Da, also known as Chinese bone setting or trauma medicine, is a traditional Chinese therapeutic practice that has been used for thousands of years. It involves the use of massage, herbal remedies, acupuncture, cupping, and other techniques to treat injuries and promote overall wellness. Becoming a Dit Da practitioner can be a rewarding career path for those interested in helping others achieve better health and well-being. Below we will discuss the steps to becoming a Dit Da practitioner.

Education and Training

The first step to becoming a Dit Da practitioner is to obtain the necessary education and training. This may involve attending a college or university that offers a degree program in traditional Chinese medicine (TCM) or attending a TCM school. Some TCM schools offer specialized programs in Dit Da that focus specifically on the treatment of injuries and trauma. These programs typically take several years to complete and include coursework in anatomy, physiology, pathology, acupuncture, herbal medicine, and other related topics.

In addition to formal education, hands-on training is also necessary to become a skilled Dit Da practitioner. This may involve attending workshops or apprenticeships with experienced practitioners to learn the techniques and theories of Dit Da.

Obtaining Certification and Licensure

After completing the necessary education and training, the next step is to obtain certification and licensure. Certification can be obtained through professional organizations such as the National Certification Commission for Acupuncture and Oriental Medicine (NCCAOM) or the American Organization for Bodywork Therapies of Asia (AOBTA).

Licensure requirements for Dit Da practitioners vary by state. Some states require practitioners to be licensed acupuncturists or massage therapists, while others may have specific requirements for bone-setting practitioners. It is important to research the specific requirements for your state and obtain the necessary licensure before practicing.

Building a Clientele

Building a clientele is a crucial part of becoming a successful Dit Da practitioner. This involves marketing your services to potential clients and building a reputation for quality care. Networking with other healthcare professionals and community organizations can also help to build a referral base.

It is important to be knowledgeable about the types of injuries and conditions that Dit Da can effectively treat and to have a clear understanding of the limitations of the practice. Good communication skills and a compassionate bedside manner are also important for building trust and rapport with clients.

Continuing Education

Continuing education is essential for staying up-to-date with the latest research, techniques, and trends in Dit Da and TCM. This may involve attending conferences, workshops, and seminars, or taking online courses.

Continuing education also helps to maintain certification and licensure requirements and demonstrates a commitment to ongoing professional development. Additionally, it can help to expand the scope of practice and offer additional services to clients.

Creating a Professional Environment

Creating a professional environment is important for building trust with clients and maintaining a successful practice. This may involve setting up a comfortable and inviting treatment room, using clean and hygienic equipment, and maintaining proper record-keeping practices.

Creating a welcoming and professional atmosphere can help to build a loyal client base and establish a reputation for quality care.

The path to becoming a professional

Dit

Da therapist

Dit Da therapy is a traditional Chinese medicine technique that involves the use of various therapeutic methods to treat a wide range of injuries and illnesses. These methods include acupuncture, herbal remedies, cupping, moxibustion, and gua sha, among others. The practice of Dit Da therapy has been passed down through generations of Chinese practitioners, and today, it is recognized as a valuable complementary therapy in many parts of the world.

If you are interested in becoming a professional Dit Da therapist, there are several paths you can take. Below we will explore some of the steps you can take to become a licensed and respected practitioner of this ancient art.

The first step to becoming a professional Dit Da therapist is to gain a solid foundation in traditional Chinese medicine. This includes a thorough understanding of the concepts of qi, yin and yang, the five elements, and the meridian system. You will also need to become proficient in the diagnostic techniques used in Chinese medicine, such as tongue diagnosis, pulse diagnosis, and palpation.

Once you have a strong foundation in traditional Chinese medicine, you can begin to focus on the specific techniques used in Dit Da therapy. This may involve additional coursework or training in acupuncture, cupping, moxibustion, gua sha, and herbal remedies. Many schools of traditional Chinese medicine offer specialized courses or certification programs in Dit Da therapy, so it is important to do your research and find a program that meets your needs.

In addition to formal training, it is also important to gain hands-on experience in the practice of Dit Da therapy. This may involve working as an apprentice or assistant to an experienced practitioner, or volunteering your time at a clinic or wellness center. By gaining practical experience in the field, you will develop a deeper understanding of the techniques used in Dit Da therapy, as well as the patient-care skills necessary to be an effective practitioner.

As you gain experience and expertise in the field of Dit Da therapy, you may choose to pursue licensure or certification as a professional practitioner. Requirements for licensure vary by state and country, but typically involve completing a certain number of training hours, passing a licensing exam, and maintaining ongoing continuing education credits. Many professional organizations and associations also offer certification programs for practitioners who meet certain criteria.

Once you have completed your training and gained the necessary experience and credentials, you can begin to establish your own practice as a professional Dit Da therapist. This may involve renting or leasing office space, building a client base through marketing and networking, and managing the administrative aspects of running a small business. It is important to stay up-to-date on the latest trends and techniques in the field, and to continue your education and training throughout your career.

Becoming a professional Dit Da therapist can be a rewarding and fulfilling career choice for those with a passion for traditional Chinese medicine and a desire to help others heal and recover from injury and illness. Whether you choose to work independently or as part of a larger healthcare team, the skills and knowledge you gain in the practice of Dit Da therapy will serve you well throughout your career.

Ethics and responsibilities of

Dit

Da practitioners

Dit Da therapy is an ancient Chinese method of treating injuries and promoting overall health and well-being. While the techniques used in this therapy are highly effective, it is important for Dit Da practitioners to adhere to a strict code of ethics and responsibilities to ensure the safety and comfort of their patients.

The first responsibility of a Dit Da practitioner is to always prioritize the well-being of their patients. This includes assessing the patient's condition and using the appropriate techniques and treatments to provide relief and promote healing. It is also important for the practitioner to keep detailed records of each patient's progress and adjust the treatment plan as necessary.

Another important ethical consideration is informed consent. Before beginning any treatment, the practitioner must fully explain the treatment plan to the patient and obtain their consent. This includes explaining the potential benefits and risks of the treatment, as well as any alternative options that may be available.

Dit Da practitioners must also maintain a high level of professionalism and confidentiality. Patients should feel comfortable sharing their personal and medical information with the practitioner, and the practitioner must keep this information confidential unless required by law to disclose it.

It is also the responsibility of the Dit Da practitioner to continue their education and stay up-to-date on the latest techniques and treatments in the field. This includes attending seminars and workshops, as well as staying informed on any changes to laws and regulations governing the practice of Dit Da therapy.

As with any medical practice, there are potential risks and complications associated with Dit Da therapy. It is the responsibility of the practitioner to fully explain these risks to the patient and take all necessary precautions to minimize them. This includes properly sterilizing equipment and maintaining a clean and safe treatment environment.

Finally, Dit Da practitioners must maintain a respectful and compassionate attitude towards their patients. This includes treating each patient with dignity and respect, and listening to their concerns and questions with empathy and understanding.

Chapter Twenty-One

Building Your Dit Da Practice

Dit Da, a traditional Chinese medicine practice, involves various therapeutic techniques to treat pain and injuries. Building a Dit Da practice requires a solid foundation in the principles of traditional Chinese medicine, knowledge of different therapeutic techniques, and a commitment to ethical practices.

To build a successful Dit Da practice, it is essential to first establish a strong foundation in traditional Chinese medicine. This includes a thorough understanding of the five elements, Yin and Yang theory, and the meridian system. A deep understanding of these principles will enable practitioners to identify imbalances in the body and understand how to restore balance and promote healing through Dit Da techniques.

Once the foundation in traditional Chinese medicine is established, the next step is to gain knowledge of different therapeutic techniques. There are numerous Dit Da techniques, including cupping, Gua Sha, acupuncture, moxibustion, herbal plasters, and liniments. Understanding the unique benefits of each technique and how they can be used to treat specific injuries and conditions is crucial in developing a comprehensive Dit Da practice.

It is also important to consider the tools and equipment needed to perform Dit Da techniques. For example, a practitioner may need cups for cupping, a Gua Sha tool, acupuncture needles, and moxibustion supplies. Investing in quality equipment is important for the safety and effectiveness of treatments.

Establishing a strong network of referrals is another crucial aspect of building a successful Dit Da practice. This can be accomplished through networking with other healthcare providers, such as acupuncturists, massage therapists, and physical therapists. Referral networks can help practitioners expand their patient base and provide comprehensive care for their patients.

In addition to building a referral network, it is important to develop a marketing strategy to attract new patients. This can include creating a website and social media presence, attending local health fairs and events, and offering free consultations or introductory treatments.

Ethics and responsibilities are essential components of any healthcare practice, including Dit Da. Practitioners must adhere to ethical practices, such as obtaining informed consent, maintaining patient confidentiality, and providing quality care. It is also important to maintain proper licensing and insurance to protect both the practitioner and patients.

Finally, continuing education is a crucial aspect of building a successful Dit Da practice. Staying up to date on the latest techniques, research, and best practices in traditional Chinese medicine will enable practitioners to provide the best possible care for their patients.

Setting up a successful

Dit

Da practice

Setting up a successful Dit Da practice can be a challenging endeavor. Dit Da is a traditional Chinese medicine practice that involves the use of various techniques, such as cupping, gua sha, acupuncture, and moxibustion, to treat a wide range of injuries and ailments. Below we will discuss some tips and strategies for building a successful Dit Da practice.

Education and Training

One of the most important steps in setting up a successful Dit Da practice is to have a solid education and training in traditional Chinese medicine. This can involve attending a reputable school or program that offers courses in acupuncture, herbal medicine, and other related fields. It is also important to obtain a license or certification in your state or country to legally practice as a Dit Da therapist.

Finding a Niche

In the world of traditional Chinese medicine, there are many different areas of focus that a practitioner can choose to specialize in. To build a successful Dit Da practice, it can be helpful to find a particular niche or area of expertise. This could be treating athletes or martial artists, addressing chronic pain, or working with elderly patients.

Building a Network

Building a network of other healthcare professionals and practitioners can be an important aspect of building a successful Dit Da practice. This can include other acupuncturists, herbalists, physical therapists, and chiropractors. These professionals can provide referrals and help to expand your practice.

Marketing and Promotion

Marketing and promoting your Dit Da practice is essential for attracting new clients and building your reputation in the community. This can involve creating a website, utilizing social media, attending networking events, and offering educational workshops or seminars. It is also important to build relationships with local media outlets, such as newspapers or radio stations, to help promote your practice.

Creating a Welcoming Environment

Creating a welcoming and comfortable environment for your clients can be crucial for building a successful Dit Da practice. This can involve creating a clean and peaceful treatment space, offering comfortable seating and lighting, and providing amenities such as tea or water. It is also important to greet your clients warmly and listen attentively to their concerns.

Offering Flexible Scheduling

Offering flexible scheduling options for your clients can be another important aspect of building a successful Dit Da practice. This could involve offering evening or weekend appointments, or providing online booking options. It is important to make it as easy as possible for your clients to schedule appointments and receive treatment.

Continuing Education

Continuing education is essential for staying up-to-date with the latest developments in the field of traditional Chinese medicine. This could involve attending conferences, workshops, or seminars, or taking online courses. It is important to continually expand your knowledge and skills to provide the best possible care for your clients.

Networking and collaborating with other practitioners

Networking and collaborating with other practitioners can be incredibly beneficial for Dit Da therapists, helping them to expand their skills, knowledge, and reach. Below we will we'll explore the advantages of networking and collaborating, as well as some strategies for building professional relationships.

One of the primary benefits of networking and collaborating with other practitioners is the opportunity to learn from one another. Different practitioners may have different specialties, techniques, or perspectives that can help to broaden your understanding of Dit Da therapy and enhance your skill set. For example, you might connect with a massage therapist who has experience working with athletes and learn some new techniques for addressing sports injuries, or you might collaborate with an acupuncturist and gain a deeper understanding of how acupuncture can complement Dit Da treatments.

Networking and collaborating can also help to build your reputation as a practitioner. By working with other professionals, you can develop a referral network and build a reputation for providing high-quality care. This can lead to an increase in clients and word-of-mouth referrals, ultimately helping to grow your practice.

So how can you start building these professional relationships? Here are a few tips:

1. Attend professional events and conferences: Attending events such as workshops, conferences, and seminars can be a great way to meet other practitioners and learn about new techniques and approaches in the field. Look for events that are relevant to your practice, and make an effort to connect with other attendees and presenters.

2. Join professional organizations: There are many professional organizations for Dit Da therapists, as well as related fields such as acupuncture

and massage therapy. These organizations can provide opportunities for networking, continuing education, and staying up-to-date on industry news and trends.

3. Volunteer or participate in community events: Participating in community events or volunteering your services can be a great way to meet other practitioners and build relationships with potential referral sources. For example, you might volunteer to provide sports massage at a local 5k race, or offer free acupuncture treatments at a health fair.

4. Connect on social media: Social media can be a powerful tool for building professional relationships, allowing you to connect with practitioners from all over the world. Look for groups or forums related to Dit Da therapy, or connect with practitioners who share your interests or specialties.

When networking and collaborating with other practitioners, it's important to maintain professional boundaries and ethics. This means respecting the scope of practice of other practitioners, not sharing confidential client information, and being transparent about your qualifications and experience.

Chapter Twenty-Two

Continuing Education and Research

Dit Da is an ancient Chinese therapy used for pain relief, healing, and prevention of injuries. The practice has evolved over the years and has become more popular in the Western world. In recent times, many practitioners have taken an interest in this form of therapy, which has resulted in more research and innovations in the field. Continuing education and research are crucial to the growth of the Dit Da practice.

Continuing education is vital for Dit Da practitioners. As with any medical practice, it is important to stay up-to-date with the latest techniques and advancements in the field. Continuing education helps practitioners improve their knowledge and skills, providing the opportunity to learn new techniques and approaches that can improve patient outcomes.

One way to continue education in Dit Da is by attending workshops and seminars. These events offer practitioners the opportunity to learn from experienced practitioners, researchers, and educators. Workshops and seminars may cover various topics related to Dit Da, such as cupping therapy, gua sha, herbal remedies, and more. Practitioners can also learn about new advancements and techniques that have been developed in the field.

Another way to continue education is by pursuing advanced degrees or certifications in related fields. For example, practitioners can obtain a degree in acupuncture, traditional Chinese medicine, or physical therapy, which can provide them with a deeper understanding of the body and its functions. Certification in massage therapy or other complementary practices can also be helpful.

Research is also essential to the growth and development of the Dit Da practice. It provides an opportunity to investigate the effectiveness of various techniques and treatments. Research can help practitioners improve their understanding of the underlying mechanisms of Dit Da therapy and its impact on the body.

Research can also help validate the effectiveness of Dit Da therapy. As more research is conducted, it can help to establish Dit Da therapy as a credible and evidence-based practice. Research can also help to identify new techniques and approaches that can be used to improve patient outcomes.

Collaboration with other practitioners is also an important aspect of continuing education and research. Working with other practitioners can provide practitioners with different perspectives and approaches to Dit Da therapy. Collaborating with other practitioners can also lead to new research opportunities, allowing practitioners to contribute to the growth and development of the field.

Staying

up-to-date

with the latest developments in

Dit

Da

Dit Da is a traditional Chinese medicine practice that has been used for centuries to treat various injuries and illnesses. As with any field, there are always new developments and advancements that practitioners need to stay up-to-date with to provide the best care possible. Below we will explore some of the ways that Dit Da practitioners can stay informed about the latest developments in the field.

One of the best ways to stay up-to-date with the latest developments in Dit Da is by continuing education. This can involve taking courses, attending conferences and workshops, and reading books and research papers. Continuing education can help practitioners learn about new techniques, tools, and treatments, as well as expand their knowledge of the underlying principles of Dit Da.

In addition to formal continuing education, practitioners can also benefit from networking and collaborating with other professionals in the field. This can involve attending local or national meetings of Dit Da associations, participating in online forums or social media groups, and reaching out to other practitioners for advice or consultation. Collaboration can help practitioners learn from each other, share experiences, and stay informed about the latest developments in the field.

Another way to stay up-to-date with the latest developments in Dit Da is by staying informed about research in the field. This can involve reading research papers and articles, as well as following the work of leading researchers and organizations. Keeping up with the latest research can help practitioners understand the evidence behind different treatments and techniques, as well as stay informed about emerging trends and innovations.

Finally, practitioners can also stay up-to-date with the latest developments in Dit Da by staying informed about the broader healthcare landscape. This can involve reading news articles and following developments in related fields, such as sports medicine, physical therapy, and pain management. Understanding how other fields are approaching similar issues can help practitioners gain new insights and ideas that they can apply to their own practice.

Research and case studies in the field of

Dit

Da

Dit Da is a traditional Chinese therapy that has been used for centuries to treat various injuries, from bruises and sprains to fractures and internal damage. Although it has been practiced for thousands of years, there is still much research to be done in the field of Dit Da, both to further our understanding of the therapy and to improve its effectiveness.

One area of research in the field of Dit Da is the use of herbs and other natural remedies in the therapy. Many Dit Da practitioners rely on herbal plasters and liniments, as well as other natural ingredients, to help reduce pain and inflammation and promote healing. Researchers are currently exploring the efficacy of these remedies, as well as the most effective ways to use them.

Another area of research in the field of Dit Da is the use of manual therapies such as cupping, Gua Sha, and moxibustion. These therapies have been used in conjunction with Dit Da for centuries, and are believed to help improve circulation and promote healing. Researchers are currently exploring the mechanisms by which these therapies work, as well as the most effective techniques for performing them.

Case studies are also an important area of research in the field of Dit Da. These studies involve analyzing the treatment of specific injuries and evaluating the effectiveness of the therapy used. Case studies can help Dit Da practitioners to better understand how the therapy can be used to treat different injuries, and to develop more effective treatment plans.

Research in the field of Dit Da is also focused on the long-term effects of the therapy. Many Dit Da practitioners believe that the therapy can help to prevent injuries and promote overall health and well-being. Researchers are exploring the mechanisms by which Dit Da may have these long-term effects, as well as the most effective ways to incorporate the therapy into a regular self-care routine.

Finally, research is also focused on the safety of Dit Da therapy. While the therapy has been used for centuries with few reported adverse effects, there is still much to be learned about the safety of the therapy and how to ensure that it is used in the most effective and safe manner possible. Researchers are exploring the potential risks associated with Dit Da, as well as ways to minimize these risks.

Chapter Twenty-Three

Resources and Further Reading

Dit Da, or "hit medicine," is an ancient Chinese therapy used to treat injuries and promote overall health and wellness. Over the years, many practitioners have written about the techniques and treatments used in Dit Da, and there are a variety of resources available for those interested in learning more about this practice.

1. One of the most comprehensive resources available is the book "Dit Da: The Essential Medicine of the Martial Arts" by Master Sunyata Saraswati. This book provides an in-depth look at the history of Dit Da, as well as detailed information on the techniques, treatments, and tools used in the practice. It also includes case studies, formulas for herbal remedies, and advice on developing a daily Dit Da practice.

Another excellent resource for those interested in Dit Da is the website www.DitDa.net. This website offers a wealth of information on the practice, including articles, videos, and a directory of Dit Da practitioners. It also features a forum where practitioners can share information and advice with each other.

For those looking for more advanced study in Dit Da, the Institute of Classical Asian Medicine in Santa Fe, New Mexico offers a comprehensive program in Dit Da and other traditional Chinese therapies. The program includes training in acupuncture, herbal medicine, and massage therapy, as well as specialized training in Dit Da techniques and treatments.

2. In addition to these resources, there are a number of books and articles available on the topic of Dit Da. Some of the most notable include "Chinese Herbal Medicine: Materia Medica" by Bensky and Gamble, "A Tooth from the Tiger's Mouth: How to Treat Your Injuries with Powerful Healing Secrets of the Great Chinese Warrior" by Tom Bisio, and "The Ancient Art of Life and Death: The Book of Dim Mak" by Dr. Jerry Alan Johnson.

Books, websites, and organizations related to

Dit

Da

Dit Da is a Chinese healing art that involves using herbal remedies, manual techniques, and other methods to treat injuries and promote healing. For those interested in learning more about this practice, there are many resources available, including books, websites, and organizations.

1. One book that is highly recommended for those interested in Dit Da is "Dit Da: The Chinese Art of Trauma Healing" by Chris Davis. This book provides a comprehensive overview of the history and principles of Dit Da, as well as detailed information on specific techniques and remedies. It also includes case studies and practical advice for those looking to incorporate Dit Da into their own healing practice.

Another useful resource for those interested in Dit Da is the website DitD a.org. This website is run by the Dit Da Institute, a non-profit organization dedicated to preserving and promoting the practice of Dit Da. The site includes articles, videos, and other resources on a wide range of topics related to Dit Da, from basic principles to advanced techniques.

There are also several organizations dedicated to promoting Dit Da and other traditional Chinese healing arts. The American Association of Oriental Medicine (AAOM) is one such organization, and it offers resources and training opportunities for those interested in this field. The National Certification Commission for Acupuncture and Oriental Medicine (NC-CAOM) is another organization that offers certification and training programs in traditional Chinese medicine, including Dit Da.

For those looking to connect with other practitioners and enthusiasts of Dit Da, there are many online forums and social media groups devoted to this practice. These communities can be a great resource for sharing knowledge, asking questions, and getting support from others who are passionate about Dit Da.

In addition to these resources, there are also many other books, websites, and organizations that can provide valuable information and support for those interested in Dit Da. Whether you are a beginner looking to learn more about the principles and techniques of this practice, or an experienced practitioner looking to expand your knowledge and skills, there are many resources available to help you on your journey.

Opportunities for advanced training and learning

Dit Da is a healing practice that has been used for centuries in traditional Chinese medicine to treat various injuries and ailments. It involves a range of techniques and remedies designed to promote healing, reduce pain, and improve overall health and well-being. For those interested in advanced training and learning in Dit Da, there are a number of opportunities available to further develop their skills and knowledge.

One of the most popular ways to advance one's knowledge of Dit Da is through workshops and seminars. These events provide the opportunity to learn from experienced practitioners and teachers who can share their expertise and insights. Workshops may cover a range of topics, including specific techniques, remedies, and treatments for different types of injuries and health conditions. Seminars may focus on broader themes related to Dit Da, such as the history and philosophy of traditional Chinese medicine, or the use of acupuncture and herbal medicine in conjunction with Dit Da.

Another option for advanced training is to pursue formal education in traditional Chinese medicine. This typically involves completing a degree or diploma program at a recognized institution. These programs may cover a range of topics related to traditional Chinese medicine, including acupuncture, herbal medicine, and massage therapy. Many programs also include courses on Dit Da and its various techniques and remedies.

In addition to formal education and workshops, there are also opportunities for self-directed learning through books, videos, and online resources. There are many books available on the topic of Dit Da, covering a range of topics such as theory, history, and practical techniques. Videos and online courses are also widely available, providing step-by-step instruction on various Dit Da techniques and remedies.

For those looking to become a professional Dit Da practitioner, there are also certification programs available. These programs typically require a certain level of education and practical experience in traditional Chinese medicine and Dit Da. Upon completion, practitioners are recognized as certified Dit Da practitioners and can practice and provide treatments with confidence and expertise.

One important consideration when pursuing advanced training and learning in Dit Da is to ensure that the sources and instructors are reputable and knowledgeable. It is important to seek out instructors and programs that have a strong foundation in traditional Chinese medicine and can provide practical and effective treatments.

In addition to advanced training and learning opportunities, there are also a number of organizations dedicated to promoting and advancing the practice of Dit Da. These organizations may provide resources and support for practitioners, as well as opportunities for networking and collaboration.

* 9 7 8 1 7 7 6 9 6 8 2 6 8 *
SD - #0051 - 140926 - C0 - 229/152/9 - PB - 9781776968268 - Matt Lamination